Treatment and Management of Allergic Rhinitis

Massoud Mahmoudi
Editor

Treatment and Management of Allergic Rhinitis

Springer

Editor
Massoud Mahmoudi, DO, PhD, FACOI, FAOCAI, FACP
Clinical Professor, Department of Medicine
University of California San Francisco
San Francisco, CA, USA

American Osteopathic College of Allergy and Immunology
Fountain Hills, AZ, USA

ISBN 978-3-031-88106-0 ISBN 978-3-031-88107-7 (eBook)
https://doi.org/10.1007/978-3-031-88107-7

This Springer imprint is published by the registered company Springer Nature Switzerland AG
The registered company address is: Gewerbestrasse 11, 6330 Cham, Switzerland

To the memory of my mother Zohreh and to my father Mohammad H. Mahmoudi, my wife Lily, and my sons Sam and Sina for their support and encouragement.

Preface

Millions of people suffer from allergic rhinitis worldwide. We, as providers, are responsible for updating our knowledge on this devastating chronic condition and utilizing it for the treatment of our patients. In the last decade we have learned more ways to treat and manage allergic rhinitis. As we continue to apply traditional modalities, we include newer therapeutic regimens to better serve the suffering patients. We believe that the approach to treatment and management of allergic rhinitis should be comprehensive. Such a wide spectrum of management should include prophylactic measures, medications, immunotherapy, and modalities which are underutilized, such as osteopathic techniques. With that in mind, I have prepared this brief, yet comprehensive collection of topics on the treatment and management of allergic rhinitis.

This book is composed of ten chapters and two parts. The first part begins with introductory chapters on anatomy and physiology of the upper respiratory system, introducing common allergens in North America and the world, and description of the allergic rhinitis. The second part of the book covers preventive measures of the disease and treatment and management. We have included chapters on osteopathic techniques utilized in treatment of rhinitis which have added to the uniqueness of this collection.

This project would not have been possible without the help and support of the editorial team and publishing staff at Springer. I would like to express my thanks to our editorial manager, Michelle Tam at Springer. And finally, I thank Richard Lansing, the editorial director of Clinical Medicine in the United States at Springer, who has been supportive of all my projects throughout the years with the publisher.

I appreciate hearing your comments and suggestions for use in what I hope to be the second edition of this title. Please contact me at allergycure@sbcglobal.net.

Los Gatos, CA, USA Massoud Mahmoudi

Contents

Contributors

Nicole Akar-Ghibril, MD Division of Immunology, Allergy, and Pediatric Rheumatology, Joe DiMaggio Children's Hospital, Memorial Healthcare System, Hollywood, FL, USA

Jonathan A. Bernstein, MD Department of Internal Medicine, Division of Rheumatology, Allergy and Immunology, Partner Advanced Allergy Services, LLC, Partner Bernstein Clinical Research Center, University of Cincinnati College of Medicine, Cincinnati, OH, USA

Shalakha Bonthu, BS Charles E. Schmidt College of Medicine, Florida Atlantic University, Boca Raton, FL, USA

Meghan Callahan, BS, MS Lake Erie College of Osteopathic Medicine, Elmira, NY, USA

Christopher Chang, MD, PhD, MBA Division of Immunology, Allergy, and Pediatric Rheumatology, Joe DiMaggio Children's Hospital, Memorial Healthcare System, Hollywood, FL, USA

Gisoo Ghaffari, MD Division of Pulmonary, Allergy and Critical Care Medicine, Pennsylvania State College of Medicine, Hershey, PA, USA

Megan E. Hanna, MD Department of Internal Medicine, University of Florida, Gainesville, FL, USA

Amna Hassan, MBBS Department of Internal Medicine, Division of Rheumatology, University of Cincinnati College of Medicine, Allergy and Immunology, Cincinnati, OH, USA

Robert W. Hostoffer, DO, LhD, MSMEd, MBA, FAAP, FACOP Cleveland Medical Center, University Hospitals, Cleveland, OH, USA
Allergy/Immunology Associates, Inc, Mayfield Heights, OH, USA

Zachary Hostoffer, DO St John Internal Medicine Residency, University Hospitals, Westlake, OH, USA

Olivia Humpel, BS Lake Erie College of Osteopathic Medicine, Bradenton, FL, USA

Jonathan Jalali Department of Medicine, David Geffen School of Medicine at UCLA, Los Angeles, CA, USA
VA Greater Los Angeles Health Care System, Los Angeles, CA, USA

Jack Jeskey Cleveland Medical Center, University Hospitals, Cleveland, OH, USA

Devi Jhaveri, DO Cleveland Medical Center, University Hospitals, Cleveland, OH, USA

Timothy Kaddis, MD Department of Medicine, David Geffen School of Medicine at UCLA, Los Angeles, CA, USA
VA Greater Los Angeles Health Care System, Los Angeles, CA, USA

Eshika Kohli, BS, OMS Lake Erie College of Osteopathic Medicine at Seton Hill, Greensburg, PA, USA

Dennis Ledford Division of Allergy and Immunology, Department of Internal Medicine, Morsani College of Medicine, University of South Florida and James A. Haley VA Hospital, Tampa, FL, USA

Massoud Mahmoudi, DO, PhD, FACOI, FAOCAI, FACP Clinical Professor, Department of Medicine, University of California San Francisco, San Francisco, CA, USA
American Osteopathic College of Allergy and Immunology, Fountain Hills, AZ, USA

Kate McDonough Allergy/Immunology Associates, Inc, Mayfield Heights, OH, USA

Ann Printy, DO Department of Medical Education, Pediatric Residency Program, Akron Children's Hospital, Akron, OH, USA

Karishma Raju, MD Department of Medicine, David Geffen School of Medicine at UCLA, Los Angeles, CA, USA
VA Greater Los Angeles Health Care System, Los Angeles, CA, USA

Lauren Reinhold, DO Cleveland Medical Center, University Hospitals, Cleveland, OH, USA

Marija J. Rowane, DO Oklahoma State University Medical Center, Tulsa, OK, USA

Remie Saab, MD Cleveland Medical Center, University Hospitals, Cleveland, OH, USA

Alyssa S. Saxton, MD Department of Internal Medicine, University of Florida, Gainesville, FL, USA

Shane Stone, DO Department of Internal Medicine-Pediatrics, Pennsylvania State College of Medicine, Hershey, PA, USA

Nicole Tierney, BA University of Northern Iowa, Cedar Falls, IA, USA

Vivian Wang, MD Department of Medicine, David Geffen School of Medicine at UCLA, Los Angeles, CA, USA
VA Greater Los Angeles Health Care System, Los Angeles, CA, USA

Jessica Wilson, DO Case Western Reserve University/ University Hospitals Cleveland Medical Center, Cleveland, OH, USA

Sarah K. Wise, MD, MSCR Department of Otolaryngology Head and Neck, Emory University, Atlanta, GA, USA

Joseph Yusin, MD Department of Medicine, David Geffen School of Medicine at UCLA, Los Angeles, CA, USA
VA Greater Los Angeles Health Care System, Los Angeles, CA, USA

Part I
Introduction

Chapter 1
Anatomy and Physiology of the Upper Respiratory System

Megan E. Hanna, Alyssa S. Saxton, Sarah K. Wise, and Dennis Ledford

Abbreviation

sIgE	Allergen-specific immunoglobulin E
AR	Allergic rhinitis
APC	Antigen-presenting cell
AMP	Antimicrobial peptide
CGRP	Calcitonin gene-related peptide
CN	Cranial nerve
CRS	Chronic rhinosinusitis
CRSwNP	Chronic rhinosinusitis with nasal polyps
GM-CSF	Granulocyte-macrophage colony-stimulating factor
Ig	Immunoglobulin
IL	Interleukin
ICA	Internal carotid artery
LT	Leukotriene
LAR	Local allergic rhinitis
NALT	Nasal-associated lymphoid tissue
NST	Nasal septal turbinate

M. E. Hanna (✉) · A. S. Saxton
Department of Internal Medicine, University of Florida, Gainesville, FL, USA
e-mail: megan.hanna@medicine.ufl.edu; alyssa.sanchez@medicine.ufl.edu

S. K. Wise
Department of Otolaryngology Head and Neck, Emory University, Atlanta, GA, USA
e-mail: skmille@emory.edu

D. Ledford
Division of Allergy and Immunology, Department of Internal Medicine, Morsani College of Medicine, University of South Florida and James A. Haley VA Hospital, Tampa, FL, USA
e-mail: dlledford@usf.edu

M. Mahmoudi (ed.), *Treatment and Management of Allergic Rhinitis*,
https://doi.org/10.1007/978-3-031-88107-7_1

PAMP	Pathogen-associated molecular pattern
PRR	Pattern recognition receptor
PAF	Platelet-activating factor
PND	Postnasal drip
PG	Prostaglandin
SP	Surfactant protein
TNF	Tumor necrosis factor
ILC2	Type 2 innate lymphoid cell
URT	Upper respiratory tract
VIP	Vasoactive intestinal peptide

Embryology and Development of the Upper Respiratory Tract

Gestational Development

The respiratory system begins to develop in the embryo at approximately week 4 of gestation. Olfactory pits, formed from ectodermal tissue of the anterior head region, invaginate and fuse with endodermal tissue of the developing pharynx. Around week 7 of gestation, the cartilaginous nasal capsule develops as two separate masses surrounding the forming nasal cavities and septum and becomes defined cartilage by the third month of gestation (Neskey et al. 2009) (Fig. 1.1).

The first paranasal sinus to arise is the maxillary sinus at weeks 11–12. The maxillary sinuses develop from the cartilaginous nasal capsule and, at week 20, extend into the ossifying maxilla bones. In week 12 the ethmoidal bulla forms; the bulla is the most prominent anterior ethmoid cell. Between weeks 16 and 20, the posterior ethmoid cells develop from the posterior aspect of the ethmoidal infundibulum. Shortly after, the sphenoid sinuses begin to develop from a small invagination of the nasal mucosal into the posterior portion of the cartilaginous nasal capsule. The last sinuses to develop are the frontal sinuses at week 12–16 (Lee et al. 2022).

Postnatal Development

Compared to adults, infants have a more vulnerable respiratory system due to anatomic and physiologic differences, including a smaller respiratory tract diameter, a tongue that nearly fills the oral cavity, decreased pharyngeal muscle tone, immature breathing control, and preferential nasal breathing. As a result, compared to older children and adults, infants have greater resistance in their URT, increasing the risk of upper airway obstruction and collapse. These limitations are compounded by a higher relative oxygen consumption requiring a more rapid respiratory rate. Other risk factors for URT obstruction include a further decrease in muscle tone during sleep with an increased time asleep and proportionally greater narrowing of the nasal passage during illness. Additionally, the infant eustachian tubes are shorter,

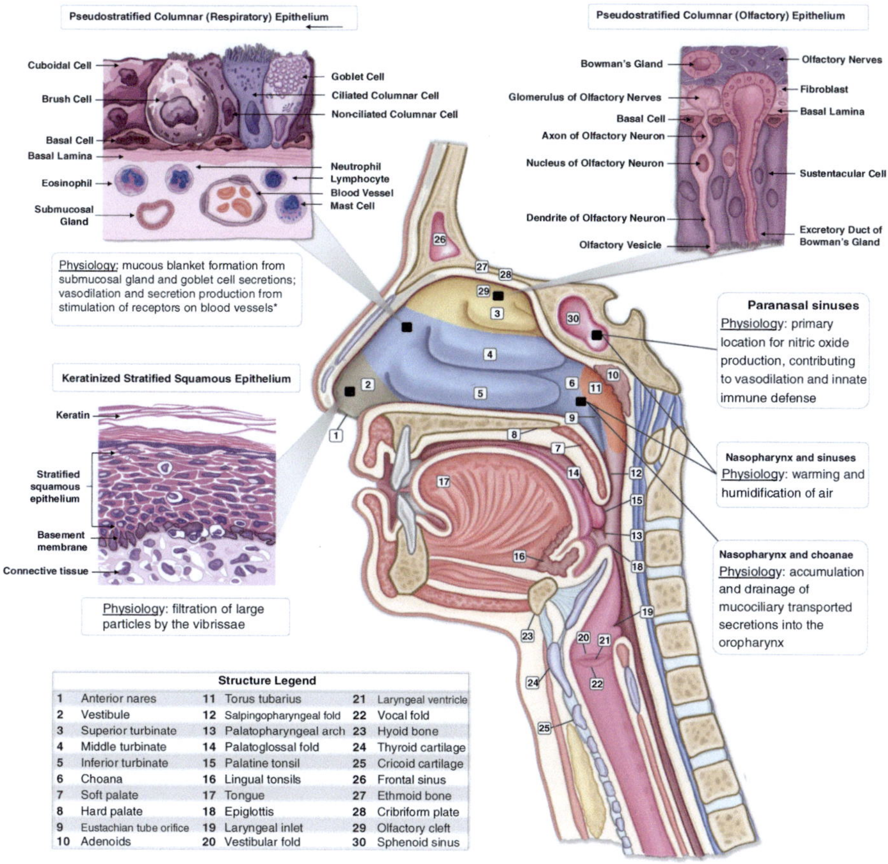

Fig. 1.1 Upper respiratory tract anatomy, histology, and physiology

more mobile, and more horizontal, resulting in reduced otic mucus drainage and increased middle ear secretions (Di Cicco et al. 2021; Trachsel et al. 2022).

Childhood Development

From infancy to early childhood, anatomical restructuring significantly changes the URT's size, shape, and mechanical and functional properties. The URT rapidly enlarges in the first 3 years of life and again during adolescence. During the first 5 years of life, the URT has more pronounced growth in the vertical and transverse/lateral dimensions than in the anteroposterior dimension (Di Cicco et al. 2021).

The paranasal sinuses have a highly variable growth pattern and undergo morphological shape changes throughout childhood. The ethmoid sinuses are the first to reach adult size at approximately the age of 12 years. The sphenoid sinuses reach

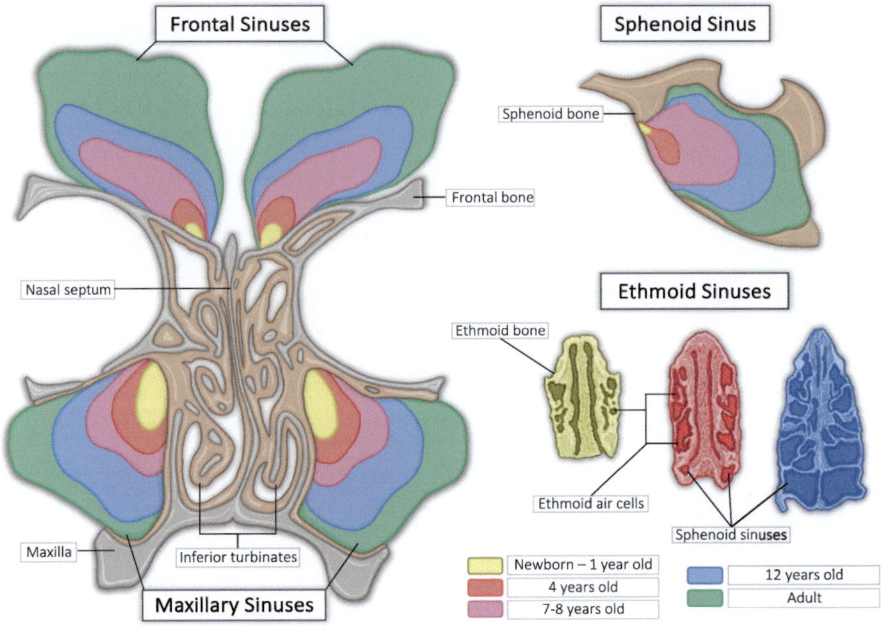

Fig. 1.2 Age-related development of the paranasal sinuses

adult size by 16 years, while the maxillary and frontal sinuses approach adult size by the age of 15–18 years (Fig. 1.2). Understanding the differences in growth and development among the sinuses is important for surgical planning in functional endoscopic sinus surgery and the interpretation of imaging studies (Lee et al. 2022).

There are several other structural variations in childhood anatomy compared with adults. Children have less efficient nasal filtration of large particles, and their eustachian tubes grow quickly but are proportionally smaller in size. The larynx is anteriorly positioned with a more complex shape. The epiglottis is relatively long, narrow, and mobile, and the Waldeyer's ring is enlarged, with rapid growth until age 5–7 years before undergoing atrophy in late childhood or early adulthood. Physiologically, like infants, children have higher metabolic rates, oxygen consumption at rest, and respiratory rates than adults (Di Cicco et al. 2021).

The Nasal Cavity

Anatomy of the Nasal Cavity

The nose and nasal cavity are composed of the external nose, the nasal vestibule, the nasal valve, the nasal septum, and turbinates (Fig. 1.1). The external nose is formed by paired nasal bones superiorly and two sets of paired cartilages inferiorly. The cartilaginous dorsum, made of paired upper lateral cartilages, shapes the middle third of the nose and supports the underlying nasal valve. The nasal tip and nostril shape are defined by the alar cartilages of lower lateral cartilages (medial, middle, and lateral crura), which attach to the upper later cartilage and the septum. Each crura is composed of two segments. The medial crus is made of the foot-plate and the columellar segments, the latter mainly responsible for nasal tip projection and the length of the nostril. The middle crus is divided into the lobule (accountable for variation in tip shape) and domal segments (contribute to the appearance of nasal tip and nostril shape). The lateral crus is the largest component among these cartilages and terminates in a chain of accessory cartilages. The nasal septum internally supports the pair of lateral cartilages.

The first portion of the URT that interacts with the external environment is the nasal vestibule. The vestibule is the only portion of the nasal cavity lined with keratinized stratified squamous epithelium and that contains thermoreceptors and vibrissae (modified hairs that filter large particles from inspired air). The nasal vestibule's epithelium transitions posteriorly to pseudostratified columnar epithelium with goblet cells, also known as the respiratory epithelium, which covers the remainder of the nasal cavity, including the sinuses. Near the squamous and respiratory epithelium junction lie the anterior nasal glands, which secrete serous mucus.

The nasal valve is immediately posterior to the nasal vestibule. It is surrounded by the superior end of the upper lateral cartilage laterally, the septum medially, and the lower rim of the pyriform aperture (bony inlet formed from nasal and maxillary bones) inferiorly (Baroody 2007). The nasal septal turbinate (NST) or 'nasal swell body' is a widened, fusiform-shaped region of erectile tissue located along the superior portion of the nasal septum. When viewing the nasal cavity, the NST is located medially and appears superior to the inferior turbinate and anterior to the middle turbinate. The NST is responsible for regulating airflow through the internal nasal valve towards the nasal turbinates and contributes to air humidification (Sahin-Yilmaz & Naclerio 2011).

The nasal septum forms the nasal midline and divides the nasal cavity into the right and left nasal cavities, or fossae. The septum has an anterior cartilaginous portion, which supports the nasal tip, and a posterior bony portion formed by the vomer and the perpendicular plate of the ethmoid bone. The superior, middle, and inferior turbinates arise from the bone of the superior and lateral nasal vault. The turbinates increase mucosal surface area, create turbulent airflow, and facilitate the impaction of larger particles onto the mucosal surface (Baroody 2007). The middle and superior turbinates also contribute to the boundaries of sinus drainage into the middle meatus (maxillary, anterior ethmoid, and frontal sinuses), superior meatus (posterior ethmoid sinus), and sphenoethmoid recess (sphenoid sinus).

Otoscopic examination of the nasal cavity allows for visualization of the vestibule, the anterior portion of the septum, the superficial vessels, the anterior portions of the middle and inferior turbinates, and any large polyps that may be present. Fiberoptic or rigid nasopharyngoscopy allows for visualization of more posterior structures of the nasal cavity: the remainder of the septum, middle meatal space and infundibulum, sphenoid ethmoid recess, middle and superior turbinates, posterior choanae, eustachian tube orifices, adenoids, nasopharynx, posterior surface of the uvula and palate,

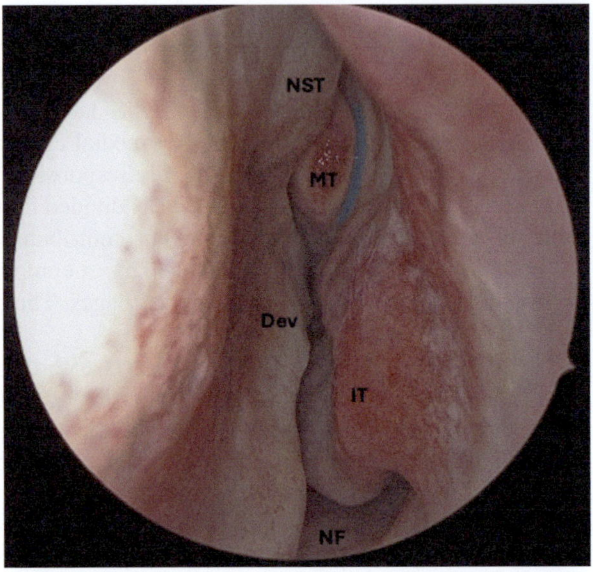

Fig. 1.3 Anterior nasal anatomy: endoscopic view of left anterior nasal cavity. The nasal septum is on the left side of the image, with nasal septal turbinate (NST) and a moderate deviation (Dev) noted. The inferior (IT) and middle turbinates (MT) are labeled, along with the nasal floor (NF). The middle meatus, lateral to the middle turbinate, is shaded in blue. This is the region where the maxillary, anterior ethmoid, and frontal sinuses drain

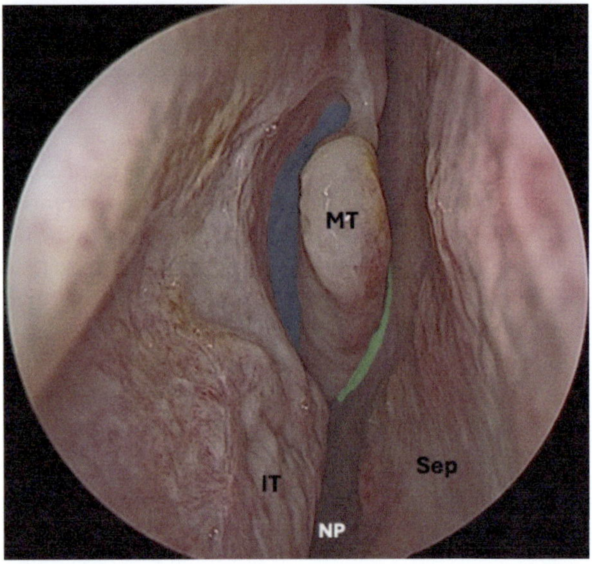

Fig. 1.4 Posterior nasal anatomy: endoscopic view of the right nasal cavity. The nasal septum is on the right side of the image (Sep). The inferior (IT) and middle turbinates (MT) are labeled, along with the nasopharynx posteriorly (NP). The middle meatus, lateral to the middle turbinate, is shaded in blue. This region is where the maxillary, anterior ethmoid and frontal sinuses drain. The region of the sphenoethmoid recess is shaded in green

velopharyngeal valve (muscular valve extending from the soft palate to the posterior pharyngeal wall separating the oral and nasal cavities), the base of the tongue, pharyngeal and lingual tonsils, vallecula, pyriform spaces, supraglottis, epiglottis, vocal folds and arytenoids, and subglottis (Anniko et al. 2010) (Figs. 1.3 and 1.4).

The histology of the nasal lining consists of an epithelial or mucosal layer overlying the submucosal layer. The mucosa is comprised of pseudostratified columnar epithelium containing ciliated and non-ciliated columnar cells with microvilli and goblet cells and infiltrating mast cells, eosinophils, and lymphocytes. Goblet cells produce secretions that contribute to a mucous blanket. The epithelial cells produce many other inflammatory and protective substances, including immunoglobulin (Ig) A secretory component. The epithelial layer is separated from the submucosa by the basement membrane. The submucosa contains blood vessels, nerves, and nasal glands.

The submucosal nasal glands, which include the anterior serous, seromucous, and Bowman glands (olfactory glands), produce most of the nasal secretions. The anterior nasal glands near the vestibule produce thin, moisturizing secretions spread by inspired air. The greatest proportion of nasal secretions are produced by seromucous glands, concentrated mainly in the anterior nasal cavity, and are either serous or mucous, depending on glandular cell type. Serous secretions are also produced by the Bowman glands, located in the lamina propria of the olfactory region. The columnar cells in the olfactory region are generally taller than those in the other respiratory epithelium (Baroody 2007).

Vasculature of the Nasal Cavity

The nasal cavity blood supply originates from branches of the internal carotid artery (ICA), including the ophthalmic artery and its branches, the anterior and posterior ethmoid arteries. The nasal cavity is also supplied by branches of the external carotid artery, including the maxillary artery and its branches the sphenopalatine artery and the greater palatine artery. These latter arteries join with the septal branch of the superior labial artery (a branch of the facial artery) in the septal portion of the vestibule, resulting in an arterial network called the Kiesselbach plexus, the most common site for epistaxis. The venous supply of the URT lies adjacent to the arterial vessels, a portion of which drains into the cavernous sinus and contributes to the intracranial spread of nasal and sinus infections. The perichondrial and periosteal arteries supply the subepithelial and glandular areas, forming a network of fenestrated capillaries that provide vascular fluid to humidify inhaled air (Baroody 2007). The nasal cavity's blood vessels contain multiple receptors that affect blood flow, vascular permeability, and secretion production. Alpha receptors are responsible for vasoconstriction of both arteries and cavernous venous vessels. Alternatively, vasodilation and increased watery secretions are achieved by stimulating beta, cholinergic, and histamine receptors (Sahin-Yilmaz & Naclerio 2011).

The lymphatic vessels from the nasal vestibule drain toward the external nose and into the subdigastric nodes, while the nasal fossa drains posteriorly into the lateral retropharyngeal nodes (Baroody 2007).

Nerve Innervation of the Nasal Cavity

The nasal cavity contains a complex neural network of sensory, parasympathetic, and sympathetic nerves that collectively regulate airflow, glandular secretion, and blood flow. The branches of the trigeminal nerve are primarily responsible for sensory innervation. Neuropeptides such as tachykinins (substance P and neurokinin A), gastrin-releasing peptides, and calcitonin gene-related peptides (CGRPs) are released by the sensory, unmyelinated, nociceptive C fibers and stimulate vasodilation and increased vascular permeability. Parasympathetic fibers originate in the midbrain, follow the path of cranial nerve (CN) seven (VII), and eventually synapse in the sphenopalatine ganglion, where they are distributed to the mucosa and submucosa. The neuropeptides, vasoactive intestinal peptide (VIP) and secretoneurin, are in the postganglionic parasympathetic fibers. Stimulation of the postganglionic fibers results in glandular secretion and vasodilation to a lesser extent.

The sympathetic fibers originate in the hypothalamus, synapse in the superior cervical ganglion (located posterior to the ICA and anterior to the cervical vertebrae 1–4), and then follow the course of the carotid plexus. Sympathetic stimulation is achieved by the interaction of norepinephrine with adrenoreceptors. Neuropeptide Y is in sympathetic neurons containing norepinephrine. With potent vasoconstricting properties, this peptide contributes to vasoconstriction and decreased nasal airway resistance.

Olfactory receptor neurons are bipolar neurons that occupy the entire thickness of the olfactory epithelium. The olfactory cilia utilize afferent nerve fibers to transmit impulses that travel through the cribriform plate of the ethmoid bone into the cranial cavity. Neural synapsis occurs with mitral cells in the olfactory bulb (located in the brain, on the ventral surface of the frontal lobe, superior to the posterior third of the cribriform plate) (Baroody 2007).

Physiology of the Nasal Cavity

The ala nasae and flaring of the nostrils increase nasal airway patency. The vestibule contributes to changes in the nasal airway resistance when its thermoreceptors are stimulated and is the most critical location for sensing nasal airflow. During inspiration, the air is directed by the nasal valve upward past the middle turbinate with an initial inspiratory velocity of roughly 18 m/second (gale force) before coursing horizontally through the central area of the nasal cavity, where the velocity slows to 2–3 m/second in adults. During expiration, the nasal valve contributes to slower airflow than in inspiration, allowing for increased air residence time and increased gas exchange at the alveoli. Overall, the nasal valve is the major source of airflow total resistance from the nasal vestibule to the pulmonary alveoli. When the cross-sectional area of the valve increases from dilator naris muscle contraction, airflow increases, and nasal flaring is observed.

After the air is inspired, laminar flow is lost, and the slower, more turbulent flow allows for rapid heat transfer and humidification of air. The air temperature reaches 34 °C, and humidity approaches 100% in the nasopharynx. As the air is expired, it is cooled, primarily by the inferior and middle turbinates. A typical adult nasal airway can conduct 20–30 liters of airflow per minute; oral breathing allows for larger volumes of air.

In adults, the nasal cycle is the alteration in airflow in which each nasal cavity varies reciprocally due to vascular engorgement of the turbinates and NST; however, the total nasal airway resistance is relatively constant. The hypothalamus and the sympathetic nervous system control the nasal cycle through deep petrosal fibers (originate in the intermediate gray horn of the spinal cord), which join with greater superficial petrosal nerve fibers and are distributed by sphenopalatine ganglion branches. Nasal congestion is medically decreased using topical nasal alpha agonists (e.g. oxymetazoline, cocaine) that cause vasoconstriction and increase nasal patency. Both the nasal septum and the turbinates contribute to the mucosal surface area of the nasal cavity and direct air toward the olfactory epithelium.

Olfactory epithelium lies along the dorsal aspect of the nasal septum, the posterior portion of the middle turbinate, and the superior portion of the superior turbinate. In the olfactory epithelium, olfaction is dependent on the bipolar neurons from the olfactory nerve (CN 1) and ophthalmic and maxillary divisions from the CN V. Like the nasal mucosa, the olfactory epithelium is covered by mucus, preventing intracranial pathogen entry through the porous cribriform plate. The olfaction process begins with odorant molecules contacting the cilia of receptor cells whose axons synapse in the olfactory bulb. Roughly 10% of airflow reaches the olfactory region; inflammatory conditions such as rhinosinusitis, viral illness, or AR can cause altered airflow and olfactory mucosal inflammation, resulting in decreased olfaction (Sahin-Yilmaz & Naclerio 2011).

Upper Respiratory Tract Immune Responses: Innate Immunity

The primary defense against infection and microorganism-induced damage to URT is innate immunity within the respiratory epithelium, which activates adaptive immunity. This occurs through mucociliary transport, microbe recognition via pattern recognition (pathogen-associated molecular patterns [PAMPs], antimicrobial peptides [AMPs]), inflammatory mediator secretion, and interactions with the adaptive immune system (Pedan et al. 2020). Sinonasal secretions and trapped particles are removed via the mucous blanket and cilia, collectively termed mucociliary transport. The mucous blanket covers the nasal cavity and consists of two phases: the sol phase (a watery periciliary layer) and the gel phase (closest to the air). The blanket is 10–15 micrometers deep and contains secretions produced by goblet cells and submucosal glands.

The mucus secretions have gel-like properties from mucins, high molecular weight glycoproteins with a protein backbone encoded by the mucin gene. The respiratory tract expresses at least 16 mucin genes, most commonly MUC5AC, MUC5B, and MUC2. The nasal valve region filters particles greater than 3 micrometers, while the nasal mucosa filters particles between 3 and 0.5 micrometers and uses ciliary flow to transport the particles to the nasopharynx. The rate of mucociliary transport ranges from 1 to 20 mm/min. Transit time is expedited by buffered hypertonic and normal saline irrigations and delayed by nasal septal deviation and CRS. Secretions are also cleared by sniffing, sneezing, and nose-blowing.

The cilia beat in a fixed direction determined by the ciliary basal foot orientation, which is similar in all cilia. Their beat consists of two strokes: the effector and the recovery stroke. During the effector stroke, the cilia straighten, encountering the gel phase and shifting the mucus. The recovery stroke follows where the cilia bend and move in the sol phase. Cilia beat faster in response to hypertonic saline and phenylephrine and slower in temperatures lower than 32 °C or above 40 °C. Mucociliary transport dysfunction compromises innate immunity, leading to colonization with pathogenic microorganisms and the development of recurrent infections (Sahin-Yilmaz & Naclerio 2011).

Secreted factors also play a role in the innate immune response. These include complement, interleukins (ILs), cytokines, nitric oxide, AMPs, and surfactant proteins (SP). Complement is responsible for host defense through opsonization, chemotaxis, and activation of leukocyte lysis of organisms, communication between innate and adaptive immunity by enhancement of antibody and immunologic memory, and immune complex and inflammatory product destruction. Cytokines IL-1β and IL-6 increase the influx of neutrophils and are observed as an inflammatory response to microorganisms in the paranasal sinus tissues. Increased nitric oxide produced by inducible nitric oxide synthase also plays a role in inflammation. Finally, bacterial endotoxins in proximity to epithelial cells result in increased permeability, alarmin release, and the formation of AMPs.

Innate immunity at the mucosal surface consists of two major cationic AMP groups: cathelicidins and defensins. Alpha defensins are found in neutrophils and nasal epithelial cells. The nasal secretions and mucosa of the paranasal sinuses contain other AMPs such as lactoferrin, lysozyme, and secretory leukoprotease inhibitors. Lysozyme is produced by serous cells of the submucosa and makes up approximately 15–30% of nasal secretion protein content. This protein prevents most airborne bacteria from colonizing the mucosa. Lactoferrin is in neutrophil granules and comprises 2–4% of nasal secretion protein content. It is bactericidal and bacteriostatic by affecting iron metabolism and assists polymorphonuclear leukocytes in binding to endothelial cells. The ciliated cells of the surface epithelium and the serous acini of the submucosal glands in the nasal mucosa contain SP-A and SP-D. These participate in the immune responses against a wide variety of bacteria, viruses, and fungi (Pedan et al. 2020).

Upper Respiratory Tract Immune Response: Pathogen Recognition

Innate and adaptive immunity differ significantly in antigen recognition. Adaptive immunity depends on T-cell and B-cell receptors, formed following exposure to the antigen and facilitated by antigen processing and presentation. Adaptive immune responses are specific to one antigen. They are not a result of a specific genetic code in germ cells and, therefore, are not transferred to the next generation. Alternatively, the innate immune receptors recognize PAMPs common to many microorganisms, such as lipopolysaccharides, lipoteichoic acid, peptidoglycan, mannans, double-stranded RNA, and free DNA. Adaptive immunity depends on antigen-presenting cells (APCs): effector cells, macrophages, dendritic cells, and respiratory epithelial cells.

The pattern recognition receptors (PRRs) on innate immune cells recognize different PAMPs and are responsible for activating T-cells. PRRs are divided into three categories: endocytic (mediating phagocytosis), signaling (mediating transcription of inflammatory cytokines and AMPs), and secreted (opsonins activating phagocytosis or complement). Additionally, nasal epithelial cells in the sinonasal tract are considered APCs and amplify the local, adaptive immune response (Pedan et al. 2020).

Upper Respiratory Tract Immune Response: Adaptive Immunity

Langerhans cells, which act as APCs, are present in the epithelium and lamina propria of the nasal mucosa. The surface epithelium contains other adaptive immune cells, such as B and T lymphocytes. The adaptive immune response recruits or modulates other cells, such as mast cells and eosinophils. Mast cells and lymphocytes (T to B cell ratio of 3:1 and T-helper [CD4] to T-effector cells [CD8] 2–3:1) increase in the lamina propria with an adaptive immune response. At rest, the nasal mucosa secretions contain IgG (2–4% of total protein), secretory (15%), non-secretory IgA (1%), and IgM secretory leukoprotease inhibitor (<1%), in addition to previously mentioned innate mucosal glycoproteins, lactoferrin, and lysozyme. IgG is found primarily at the basement membrane, preventing epithelial microorganisms from progressing into deeper layers. An increase in vascular permeability can increase the IgG mucous concentration up to 125 times. Secretory IgA is abundant in nasal secretions and binds microorganisms to prevent initial mucosal invasion.

Nasal-associated lymphoid tissue (NALT) is located throughout the nasal submucosa and is functionally analogous to Waldeyer's ring. It is an essential location for antigen-specific immune responses and activation of immunocompetent cells (B and T-cell responses and plasma cell generation). Its structure contains antigen- and microbe-retaining crypts, allowing for polyclonal activation for interaction among antigen-presenting and responding cells and for developing enhanced B-cell diversity and memory. NALT has been a research target of intranasal vaccines to elicit T-cell immunity because of its importance in the respiratory immune response (Pedan et al. 2020).

Age-Related Effects on Nasal Physiology

Several structural changes in the URT occur with aging. Collagen fiber atrophy, nasal columella retraction, and weakening of the fibrous connective tissue of the lateral cartilages and septal cartilage lead to a dropped nasal tip. As a result, the nasal airway is narrowed, airflow is decreased, and nasal congestion is more prevalent in older adults than younger adults. Nasal mucosal changes, such as atrophy and decreased blood flow, also occur with normal aging. Consequently, the nasal passages have a reduced capacity for humidification, resulting in susceptibility to dryness and irritation. With aging, the development of rhinitis is attributed to a combination of excessively thick nasal mucus due to changes in visco-elastic properties of the mucus and a decline in mucociliary transport. These age-related changes and increased cholinergic activity with aging increase the sensation of postnasal drip (PND). Lastly, olfaction and the ability to distinguish smells decrease, particularly after the seventh decade of life (Önerci 2013).

Other Conditions Affecting Nasal Physiology

Primarily affecting the central nasal cavity (posterior nasal septum, middle and superior turbinates) and subsequently the sinuses in advanced cases, central compartment atopic disease (CCAD) is a specific variant of nasal polyps. CCAD is notable for a high prevalence of allergy and low prevalence of asthma in early observational reports. CCAD may occur in AR patients with long-term exposure to inhaled allergens, even at subclinical levels (Marcus et al. 2020).

Abnormal mucociliary clearance is also a hallmark of cystic fibrosis (CF) and primary ciliary dyskinesia, predisposing affected individuals to CRS and PND. In CF, mucus viscosity is increased due to a mutation in the cystic fibrosis transmembrane conductance receptor (CFTR) gene, resulting in decreased function of the transmembrane chloride transporter. Ciliary movement is impaired further by increased mucus viscosity due to elevated levels of MUC5AC and MUC5B. In primary ciliary dyskinesia, various genetic mutations result in dysfunction or complete absence of cilia (Önerci 2013) (Table 1.1).

Nasal physiology is also disrupted in autoimmune conditions. Relapsing polychondritis is a rare condition with recurrent cartilaginous inflammation of the auricular, nasal, and tracheal cartilage. The mechanism is believed to be autoimmunity specific for the main constituent of cartilage proteoglycan. Cartilage destruction occurs from macrophage-released proteolytic enzymes metalloproteinase (MMP-3) and cathepsin L and K. Nasal chondritis is seen in roughly 25% of cases. Sjogren's syndrome is an autoimmune condition characterized by exocrine gland dysfunction and destruction. Manifestations of nasal involvement include mucosal atrophy and dryness, mucociliary dysfunction prolonging mucociliary transport time, hyposmia, hypogeusia, and nasal septal perforation (Anniko et al. 2010). Other nasal cavity conditions include nasal valve collapse, deviated septum, septal perforation, turbinate hypertrophy, concha bullosa, and paradoxical middle turbinate (Anniko et al. 2010; Önerci 2013) (Table 1.2).

Table 1.1 Pathologies and symptoms associated with each type of nasal cavity epithelium

Epithelium type	Pathology	Symptoms
Keratinized stratified squamous	Nasal obstruction and impaired nasal airflow patency from increased mucus production, inflammation, and vasodilation Increased susceptibility to epithelial atrophy from corticosteroid use	Nasal pruritis and irritation Sneezing Bleeding with corticosteroid use
Pseudostratified columnar (respiratory)	Allergen exposure, deposition, and epithelial damage with type II inflammation Proliferation of inflammatory epithelial cells (mast cells, basophils) with resultant increased vascular permeability and epithelial barrier compromise Impaired mucociliary clearance in conditions such as cystic fibrosis, primary ciliary dyskinesia, and Sjogren's syndrome	Nasal congestion from inflammation, mucus production, and decreased airflow Rhinorrhea from mucosal gland hypersecretion Polyp formation from chronic inflammation
Pseudostratified Columnar (olfactory)	Decreased airflow, nasal passage obstruction and inflammation at the olfactory cleft Olfactory sensory neurogenesis inhibition from chronic inflammation and mucus hypersecretion	Hyposmia, or decreased ability to sense and differentiate odors

Table 1.2 Pathologies and clinical manifestations associated with key anatomical structures of the nasal cavity

Key anatomy	Important physiology	Clinical pathology	Pathologic symptoms
Nasal cartilage	Provides structure and support for the anterior nasal cavity	*Relapsing polychondritis:* recurrent episodes of auricular, nasal, and tracheal cartilage inflammation; thought to be caused by autoimmunity against proteoglycan, cartilage destruction mediated by macrophages	Nasal chondritis (pain and tenderness of nose, rhinorrhea, epistaxis, saddle nose deformity), hoarseness if laryngeal cartilage is involved
Nasal septum	Separates right and left nasal cavities, regulates airflow, dorsally supports nose, maintains nasal tip/columella shape	*Deviated septum*: septum displaced away from midline; may be present at birth, can be caused by facial trauma or surgery	Unilateral nasal obstruction with difficulty breathing through the nose, epistaxis
		Septal perforation: anterior most common; can result from trauma, surgery, epistaxis cautery, nasal cocaine use, intranasal steroids, and conditions such as sarcoidosis and granulomatosis with polyangiitis	Sensation of nasal obstruction, thick rhinorrhea, saddle nose, epistaxis, whistling with inhalation

(continued)

Table 1.2 (continued)

Key anatomy	Important physiology	Clinical pathology	Pathologic symptoms
Nasal turbinates (nasal concha)	Warms and humidifies air, regulates airflow, and creates turbulence allowing for pathogen trapping, increases mucosal surface area of the nasal cavity	*Central compartment syndrome*: CRSwNP variant; MT, ST, and SNS polypoid change, associated with inflammation, allergic sensitization	Nasal congestion, rhinorrhea, hyposmia; other symptoms of AR
		Concha bullosa: pneumatized cavity usually seen in the middle turbinate; etiology unclear, though frequently concomitant with septum deviation	If large, may cause nasal obstruction, recurrent rhinosinusitis
		Paradoxical middle turbinate: inferomedially curved MT edge with concave surface facing nasal septum	Typically asymptomatic; if severe, may cause alteration in nasal airflow
		Turbinate hypertrophy: enlargement of the IT; can be caused by AR, non-AR, rhinitis medicamentoda, environmental irritants, hormonal changes	Nasal congestion worse when lying down, dry mouth and throat, improves with application of nasal decongestants
Nasal valve	Controls airflow, filters air during inhalation	*Nasal valve collapse:* weakening, narrowing or inward collapse; can be caused by aging, facial trauma, surgery (rhinoplasty)	Nasal obstruction, mouth breathing during the day

Abbreviations: *AR* allergic rhinitis, *CRSwNP* chronic rhinosinusitis with nasal polyps, *IT* inferior turbinate, *MT* middle turbinate, *SNS* superior nasal septum, *ST* superior turbinate

The Sinuses

Anatomy and Histology of the Sinuses

There are four paired paranasal sinuses: maxillary, frontal, ethmoid, and sphenoid. Mucus-producing, ciliated, pseudostratified columnar epithelium lines all the sinus cavities. The maxillary sinuses, residing in the maxillary bones beneath the eyes, are the largest and are anterior to the pterygopalatine fossa. The medial wall separates the nasal cavity from this sinus with communication through the sinus ostium opening in the middle meatus inferior to the middle turbinate. A fine layer of compact bone separates the sinus floor from the apices of the posterior maxillary teeth. Near the ostium, there is an increased number of cilia to propagate secretions upwards toward the ostium.

The frontal sinuses are typically pyramidally shaped and lie superior to the orbit within the frontal bone. The inter-frontal sinus septum divides the frontal sinus into two cavities, although variability occurs, and several septa may be present. Each frontal sinus cavity develops independently, frequently resulting in asymmetry. Consequently, the septum may deviate from the midline and away from the larger sinus. The frontal sinus drains through the ostium into the frontal recess below and eventually reaches the middle meatus lateral to the middle turbinate. The frontal recess, below the frontal sinus ostium, is surrounded by the agger nasi cells anteriorly, lamina papyracea laterally, and the middle turbinate medially. Agger nasi cells located in the anterior portion of the frontal recess are frequently present and may contribute to impaired frontal sinus drainage. Overall, the frontal sinus has the longest, most complex, and variable drainage pathway among the paranasal sinuses, increasing the risk of complicated infections. Obstruction of the frontal recess is responsible for most cases of frontal sinusitis (Baroody 2007; Anniko et al. 2010).

The sphenoid sinuses are located within the sphenoid bone, superior and posterior to the URT. Adjacent to these sinuses are the ICA and the cavernous sinuses laterally and the pituitary gland superiorly. Drainage travels from the sphenoid ostium into the sphenoethmoidal recess medial to the superior turbinate.

The ethmoid sinuses are located between the eyes and the nose and are formed from several air cells. Agger nasi cells are present in these sinuses and lie most anteriorly, with their posterior wall forming the anterior aspect of the frontal recess. The largest of the anterior ethmoid cells is the ethmoid bulla, which is attached laterally to the lamina papyracea and forms the medial wall of the orbit. The anterior ethmoid sinuses are in close proximity to the frontal and maxillary sinus ostia; therefore, disease affecting the ethmoid sinuses may secondarily impair drainage from the frontal and maxillary sinuses. Clinically, ethmoid sinus involvement is frequently observed in the setting of frontal or maxillary sinus disease (Baroody 2007). The posterior ethmoid air cells drain lateral to the superior turbinate into the superior meatus.

The most common variations in the anatomy of the nasal cavity and paranasal sinuses include agger nasi cells, nasal septal deviation, concha bullosa of the middle turbinates, variations in the superior attachment of the uncinate process, presence of a paradoxical middle turbinate, presence of Haller, Onodi, and supraorbital ethmoid cells, variations in the height of the ethmoid roof, and the formation of accessory ostia in the maxillary sinus (Anniko et al. 2010).

Vasculature and Nerve Innervation of the Sinuses

The blood supply and innervation of the maxillary sinus are comprised of branches of the maxillary artery and nerve (a branch of the trigeminal nerve). The supratrochlear and supraorbital arteries and nerves supply blood and innervation to the frontal sinus. The sphenoid sinus is supplied by the sphenopalatine artery and is innervated by the sphenopalatine nerve, comprising the parasympathetic fibers and CN V2. The anterior and posterior ethmoid arteries, branching from the ophthalmic artery, supply blood to the ethmoid sinus, while innervation is achieved by the anterior and posterior ethmoid nerves. The maxillary and ethmoid veins drain these sinuses and may affect the cavernous sinus and ophthalmic vein, which are in close proximity to the CNS and the eye (Baroody 2007).

Physiology of the Sinuses

The paranasal sinuses have multiple roles, including humidifying and heating inspired air, insulating sensitive structures from rapid temperature changes in the nose, decreasing the weight of the skull, increasing voice resonance, providing a buffer against facial trauma, and participating in immunological defense. Like the nasal cavity, the sinuses regulate mucociliary clearance via nasal secretions. These secretions are moved by cilia toward the primary natural opening, which may require transport against gravity. Similar to the nasal mucosa, the sinus mucosa shares many of the innate and adaptive immune responses described previously, including pathogen recognition and cellular host defenses. Additionally, the sinuses are the primary location for nitric oxide production in the URT and exhibit antibacterial and antiviral properties due to innate and adaptive immune responses (Anniko et al. 2010; Önerci 2013).

Clinically, inflammation of the nasal cavity may be associated with inflammation of the sinuses. Consequently, the natural narrowing at the ostia is predisposed to potential obstruction following viral infection and allergic inflammation. Barometric pressure changes may affect the sinuses if the ostia patency does not allow pressure normalization, also resulting in possible sinus obstruction. Thus, the underlying causes of sinusitis are numerous, and many overlap with the causes of rhinitis (Önerci 2013).

In addition to acute and chronic rhinosinusitis, other clinically significant conditions involving the sinuses include odontogenic sinusitis, nasal polyps (allergic, eosinophilic non-allergic, neutrophilic associated with immotile cilia and CF), inverted papilloma, mucoceles, fungal rhinosinusitis, mucus retention cysts, eosinophilic granulomatosis with polyangiitis (Churg Strauss vasculitis), granulomatosis with polyangiitis (Wegener's vasculitis), frontal recess obstruction, malignancies (most commonly squamous cell carcinoma and adenocarcinoma), and others (Anniko et al. 2010) (Table 1.3).

Table 1.3 Pathologies and clinical manifestations associated with key anatomical structures of the sinuses

Key anatomy	Important physiology	Clinical pathology	Pathologic symptoms
Frontal recess	Funnel-shaped, inward opening allowing frontal sinus drainage	*Frontal recess obstruction:* frontal sinus blockage and sinusitis; can be caused by polyps, trauma, acute infection, chronic inflammation, presence of agger nasi cells, frontal cells, or scar tissue	Purulent nasal drainage, nasal obstruction or congestion, forehead pressure or fullness, PND, fever
Paranasal sinuses	Warms and humidifies air, insulates nasal cavity, immunologic defense, buffer to facial trauma, increases vocal resonance, reduces skull weight	*Acute rhinosinusitis:* mucosa inflammation with thickened mucus, drainage, obstruction, and ciliary impairment; usually seen with URI	Lasts <4 weeks; purulent nasal drainage, facial pressure or fullness, PND, hyposmia, fever
		Chronic rhinosinusitis: chronic mucosal inflammation; AR, asthma, and nasal polyps are frequently associated with CRS	Nasal obstruction or congestion with anterior or posterior drainage, facial pressure, hyposmia
		Eosinophilic granulomatosis with polyangiitis (Churg Strauss): necrotizing vasculitis with eosinophil-mediated inflammation; initial allergic phase characterized by asthma, rhinosinusitis, nasal polyposis	Rhinorrhea, sneezing, nasal crusting, mucoid nasal discharge, eye irritation; other classic respiratory, rheumatologic, and skin findings
		Fungal rhinosinusitis: invasive infections (AIRS, CIRS, GIFS) in immunosuppressed hosts; non-invasive forms (AFRS, mycetoma, SFC) occur without immune compromise; mycetoma and SFC are often asymptomatic	Nasal congestion, facial pressure, thick nasal drainage; invasive infections may result in fever, cranial neuropathies, orbital symptoms, and mental status changes
		Granulomatosis with polyangiitis (Wegener's): small-vessel vasculitis with coagulative necrosis, granuloma formation, chronic sino-nasal inflammation; may lead to NSP, loss of turbinate, nasal bridge collapse	Rhinorrhea, purulent nasal discharge and crusting, epistaxis, otitis media; late: septal perforation, saddle nose; other classic lung, renal manifestations
		Inverted papilloma: fingerlike, inward projections; associated with chronic inflammation, HPV, EBV; benign tumor with 5-10% chance of malignant transformation	Unilateral nasal obstruction or congestion, rhinorrhea, epistaxis, hyposmia
		Mucocele: epithelial-lined cystic masses commonly occurring in frontal and ethmoid sinuses; usually caused by sinus ostia obstruction with complete sinus opacification and expansion of the bony sinus walls	Facial pressure/deformity, nasal obstruction and congestion, ophthalmic symptoms (diplopia, proptosis, ptosis)
		Mucus retention cysts: collections of mucus resulting from blocked seromucous glands of maxillary sinus; typically asymptomatic	Usually self-limiting; if symptomatic, may cause facial pressure and (rarely) recurrent sinusitis
		Nasal polyps: soft hyperplastic growths of nasal mucosal lining; caused by chronic inflammation; associated with CRS, asthma, AERD, AFRS, and CF	Nasal congestion and obstruction, mucoid rhinorrhea, hyposmia or anosmia, PND
		Odontogenic sinusitis: maxillary sinus inflammation due to infection (periodontal disease) or dental trauma of the neighboring teeth	Facial and dental pain or pressure, purulent rhinorrhea, PND, cacosmia

Abbreviations: *AERD* aspirin-exacerbated respiratory disease, *AFRS* allergic fungal rhinosinusitis, *AIRS* acute invasive rhinosinusitis, *AR* allergic rhinitis, *CF* cystic fibrosis, *CIRS* chronic invasive rhinosinusitis, *CRS* chronic rhinosinusitis, *EBV* Epstein-Barr virus, *GIFS* granulomatous invasive fungal sinusitis, *HPV* human papillomavirus, *NSD* nasal septal deviation, *NSP* nasal septal perforation, *PND* postnasal drip, *SFC* saprophytic fungal colonization, *URI* upper respiratory infection

The Nasopharynx and Oropharynx

Anatomy and Histology of the Nasopharynx

Also known as the rhino-pharynx, the nasopharynx connects the nasal cavity to the oropharynx. Its anatomic boundaries include the skull base superiorly, the soft palate inferiorly, the nasal cavity anteriorly, the posterior pharyngeal wall posteriorly, and the medial pterygoid plates and the superior pharyngeal constrictor muscles laterally (Belafsky & Lintzenich 2013). Within this structure are the eustachian tube opening, the torus tuberius, the fossa of Rosenmuller, and the adenoids (Anniko et al. 2010; Belafsky & Lintzenich 2013).

Vasculature and Nerve Innervation of the Nasopharynx

The blood supply to the nasopharynx arises from the ICA, the maxillary artery, the facial artery, and the ascending pharyngeal artery. Venous drainage occurs from the parapharyngeal venous plexus into the retropharyngeal and facial veins and, ultimately, the internal jugular vein. Lymphatic drainage begins with a capillary network in the mucosal membranes, draining eventually into the internal jugular nodes.

The anterior portion of the nasopharynx has sensory innervation from the maxillary branch of the trigeminal nerve (CN V2), while the posterior portion is innervated by the glossopharyngeal nerve (CN IX). The vagus nerve (CN X) supplies motor innervation for the muscles in the nasopharynx other than the tensor veli palatini muscle, innervated by the mandibular branch of the trigeminal nerve (CN V3), and the stylopharyngeus muscle, innervated by the glossopharyngeal nerve (CN IX) (Belafsky & Lintzenich 2013).

Musculature of the Nasopharynx and Variations in Anatomy

The nasopharyngeal muscles that originate from the eustachian tube opening include the tensor veli palatini, which tenses the soft palate, the levator veli palatini, which elevates the soft palate, and the salpingopharyngeus which elevates the pharynx. The eustachian tube orifice is opened during swallowing by all three of these muscles, which allows for the equilibration of atmospheric pressure between the middle ear cavity and the nasopharynx. Other muscles of the nasopharynx include the constrictor muscles (superior, middle, inferior, and cricopharyngeus) and the longitudinal muscles (stylopharyngeus, palatopharyngeus, and salpingopharyngeus) (Pedan et al. 2020).

Variations in the anatomy of the pharynx include the nasopharynx dimensions, superficial landmark asymmetries such as eustachian tube openings, and variations in musculature attachments (Belafsky & Lintzenich 2013).

Anatomy and Histology of the Oropharynx

The oropharynx is inferior to the nasopharynx, posterior to the oral cavity, and immediately superior to the larynx and hypopharynx, serving as a passageway for food, liquid, and air. This region spans from the soft and hard palate to the hyoid bone and the superior border of the epiglottis. The posterior one-third of the tongue, the lingual tonsils (lymphoid tissue at the base of the tongue), and the palatine tonsils (tonsils visible in oral examination) are contained within the oropharynx.

The tonsillar fossa is a triangular space created by the palatoglossal arch posteriorly and the palatopharyngeal arch anteriorly. Additionally, an aggregate of lymphoid tissue called the Waldeyer's ring is situated at the junction of the nasopharynx and oropharynx. It is comprised of the paired palatine, adenoid, and lingual tonsils. The Waldeyer's ring is an important area of immune response to inhaled or ingested antigens.

The ascending palatine branch and the facial artery (CN VII) provide the vascular supply to this area. The glossopharyngeal nerve (CN IX) supplies the sensory innervation. Like the nasopharynx, motor innervation is supplied by the vagus nerve (CN X) (Anniko et al. 2010; Belafsky & Lintzenich 2013).

Physiology of the Nasopharynx and the Oropharynx

The nasopharynx controls the eustachian tube opening via intrinsic muscles and contributes to phonation and resonance. Additionally, through mucociliary clearance, this tissue allows for transporting and draining trapped pathogens into the oropharynx. The oropharynx assists with swallowing, contributes to phonation, and allows air passage into the larynx (Anniko et al. 2010).

PND is a frequent symptom in patients with rhinitis and sinusitis. Individuals with PND usually complain of the sensation of mucus accumulating in the nasopharynx and descending into the posterior pharynx. There are several theories regarding the etiology of PND, including increased mucus viscosity, impaired ciliary function, increased secretion volume, irritant sensation from inflammation, and laryngeal edema from laryngopharyngeal reflux (LPR). PND is associated with many conditions, including AR, nonallergic rhinitis, acute and chronic rhinosinusitis, mouth breathing due to nasal congestion, and LPR in GERD (Smallwood et al. 2024).

Other conditions and pathology that affect the function of the nasopharynx include squamous carcinoma, lymphoma, adenoid hypertrophy, nasopharyngeal stenosis, nasopharyngitis, and Tornwaldt's bursa (cyst in adenoid). Conditions involving the oropharynx include Langerhans cell histiocytosis, oropharyngeal dysphagia, pharyngitis, and neuromuscular disorders (e.g. cerebrovascular accidents, amyotrophic lateral sclerosis, myasthenia gravis, dystonia) (Table 1.4) (Anniko et al. 2010).

Table 1.4 Pathologies and clinical manifestations associated with key anatomical structures of the nasopharynx and oropharynx

Key anatomy	Important physiology	Clinical pathology	Pathologic symptoms
Nasopharynx	Connects nasal cavity to the oropharynx allowing for drainage of mucociliary clearance, controls eustachian tube opening via intrinsic muscles, contributes to phonation and resonance, filters air	*Nasopharyngeal adenoid hypertrophy:* adenoid enlargement with nasal passage obstruction commonly in children; associated with infection, GERD, smoking, pollution, and allergic rhinitis	Nasal obstruction, snoring, sleep apnea, halitosis, eustachian tube blockage (otitis media), conductive hearing loss
		Nasopharyngeal stenosis: nasopharyngeal narrowing from scar tissue obstructing oropharynx communication; caused by infection (syphilis, TB, diphtheria), autoimmune disease (cicatricial pemphigoid), surgery, radiation	Rhinorrhea, nasal obstruction, snoring, sleep apnea, hyponasal speech, dysphagia, otalgia, hyposmia
		Nasopharyngitis: nasopharyngeal inflammation typically from viral URI	Cough, itchy/watery eyes, headache, sore throat
		Postnasal drip: sensation of mucus descending into posterior pharynx; may be caused by increased mucus viscosity or volume, impaired ciliary function, heightened irritant sensation from laryngo-esophageal edema	Sensation of mucus dripping or accumulating in the throat, cough (worse at night), constant need to clear throat, hoarseness, halitosis
		Tornwaldt's bursa: rare, benign mucosal cyst at nasopharyngeal midline, representing notochord communication during development; usually asymptomatic, but may become infected (termed Tornwaldt's disease)	Occipital headache, halitosis, purulent discharge into the mouth (choanal), acute otitis media and changes in hearing from eustachian tube blockage
Oropharynx	Connects nasopharynx to larynx, assists with swallowing, contributes to phonation, allows for air passage into larynx	*Langerhans cell histiocytosis*: hematologic disorder most common in children with abnormal dendritic cell proliferation and migration; may involve the oral cavity with gingival, hard palate and mandible ulceration	Facial swelling and pain, mouth pain due to oral mucosal ulceration, gingival swelling, tooth hypermobility, lymphadenopathy
		Oropharyngeal dysphagia: impaired swallowing and transfer of food; can be structural (pharyngoesophageal diverticulum, surgery), neurogenic (stroke, TBI), neuromuscular (MG), inflammatory (EOE, GERD, polymyositis)	Nasopharyngeal regurgitation, coughing, throat clearing, breathlessness with eating and drinking, sensation of "stuck" food, aspiration or choking
		Pharyngitis: inflammation of oropharyngeal mucosa; caused by URI (mononucleosis, strep throat from GAS), allergies, GERD	Infectious: sore throat, odynophagia, headache, LAD, tonsillar exudates, fever, fatigue, myalgias

Abbreviations: *EOE* eosinophilic esophagitis, *GAS* group A streptococcus, *GERD* gastroesophageal reflux disease, *LAD* lymphadenopathy, *MG* myasthenia gravis, *TB* tuberculosis, *TBI* traumatic brain injury, *URI* upper respiratory infection

The Larynx

Anatomy of the Larynx

The larynx connects the pharynx to the cervical trachea and separates the upper aerodigestive tract from the tracheobronchial tree. The larynx is composed of a cartilaginous skeleton consisting of nine cartilages (three unpaired and three paired), including the epiglottis and the thyroid, cricoid, arytenoid, corniculate, and cuneiform cartilages. The thyroid cartilage is vertical and anterior to the true and false vocal folds, protecting and supporting the vocal folds. The cricoid cartilage is in the inferior portion of the larynx, completely encircling the trachea. The arytenoid cartilages, a pair of small, pyramid-shaped structures, sit over the posterior portion of the cricoid cartilages and are joined by the corniculate cartilages of Santorini. Each cartilage base possesses vocal and muscular processes. The true vocal folds (vocal cords) are connected to the arytenoid cartilages, and rotation of the cartilages allows the vocal folds to adduct and abduct.

The epiglottis, an elastic cartilaginous flap anchored to the internal surface of the thyroid cartilage, can fold over the larynx and, along with the posterior and inferior position of the tongue, is important in excluding liquids and solids from the airway when swallowing. The vocal folds and the lateral aspects of the epiglottis are supported by the cuneiform cartilages, which are elongated, fibrous structures located in the aryepiglottic fold.

Joints between the laryngeal cartilages allow for movement, and extrinsic and intrinsic ligaments achieve stability. The laryngeal cavity is divided into three sections: supraglottic, glottic, and infraglotic. The glottic space is comprised of the vocal folds, the glottis, and the larynx ventricles.

Variations in the anatomy of the larynx include gender-related structural differences, alternate pathways for laryngeal innervation, and variations in the recurrent laryngeal nerve and its relationship with the inferior thyroid artery (Anniko et al. 2010).

Vasculature, Nerve Innervation, and Physiology of the Larynx

The larynx receives its blood supply from the superior and inferior laryngeal arteries. Venous drainage in this area travels from the superior and inferior laryngeal veins into the superior and inferior thyroid veins and finally into the internal jugular and subclavian veins. Lymphatic drainage consists of the supraglottic lymphatic nodes draining into the deep cervical lymph node chain, the supraglottic lymphatics draining into the pre- and paratracheal lymph nodes, and the laryngeal nodes, eventually draining into the lower deep cervical lymph nodes.

Nerve innervation of the larynx is supplied by CN X branches: the superior, inferior, and recurrent laryngeal nerves. The mucous membrane surrounding the laryngeal entrance is innervated by the internal branch of the superior laryngeal nerve. Laryngeal intrinsic muscles are innervated by the recurrent laryngeal nerve, apart from the cricothyroid muscle, which is innervated by the external branch of the superior laryngeal nerve.

The striated laryngeal muscles are composed of intrinsic muscles, responsible for phonation, and extrinsic muscles, which allow for laryngeal movement (Pedan et al. 2020). The larynx protects the lower respiratory tract from aspiration, assists in respiration, and contributes to phonation via the vocal folds. Conditions affecting this area include laryngitis (infectious, contact, mechanical, and allergic), laryngeal papillomatosis, squamous carcinoma, laryngopharyngeal reflux, laryngotracheal stenosis, vocal cord cysts, nodules and polyps, laryngeal nerve paralysis (vocal cord paralysis), and laryngeal cancer (most commonly squamous cell carcinoma) (Anniko et al. 2010) (Table 1.5).

Table 1.5 Pathologies and clinical manifestations associated with key anatomical structures of the larynx

Key anatomy	Important physiology	Clinical pathology	Pathologic symptoms
Larynx (entire region)	Connects the pharynx to the cervical trachea, separates the upper aerodigestive tract from the tracheobronchial tree, prevents food entry into the trachea, assists with cough reflex, ventilation, and widens the airway during respiration	*Laryngeal papillomatosis:* exophytic wart-like tumors that can extend from the nasal cavity to the lungs; caused by human papillomavirus (HPV)	Hoarseness, chronic cough, dysphagia, apneic episodes, difficulty breathing, increased vocal effort
		Laryngitis: inflammation caused by URI, vocal trauma, irritants (dust, fumes, allergens, smoke), GERD, asthma, and autoimmune disorders	Hoarseness, early vocal fatigue, dry cough, throat clearing, sore or dry throat with thick mucus
		Laryngopharyngeal reflux: reflux of stomach contents onto the glottis and vocal cords; associated with inappropriate relaxation of the UES	Hoarseness, globus sensation, cough after eating or lying down, PND, regurgitation or choking
		Laryngotracheal stenosis: laryngeal scarring and narrowing below the level of vocal cords; caused by trauma, intubation, infections (syphilis, leprosy, diphtheria, TB), vasculitic or granulomatous conditions (GPA, sarcoidosis), neoplasms, congenital defect	Respiratory compromise, high-pitched and noisy breathing (stridor), difficulty exhaling, coughing, throat clearing, hoarseness, weak voice

(continued)

Table 1.5 (continued)

Key anatomy	Important physiology	Clinical pathology	Pathologic symptoms
Vocal cords	Adduct, abduct, and vibrate to result in production of voice	*Laryngeal nerve paralysis:* vocal cord paralysis, usually unilateral; caused by neck or surgical trauma (thyroid surgery, carotid endarterectomy), neurological disease (stroke, MS, CNS tumors), idiopathic; may be associated with pathology in the chest when it occurs on the left side due to intrathoracic course of recurrent laryngeal nerve	Change in vocal pitch and volume, stridor, shortness of breath, noisy breathing, dysphagia, choking or coughing while eating
		Vocal cord cysts: benign, fluid-filled or semisolid sacs medially located; can present in utero or develop with voice overuse or glandular duct irritation	Hoarseness, voice strain, change quality of voice, pitch limitations, pain with speaking or singing
		Vocal cord nodules: small, benign symmetrical masses of vocal cords; usually caused by voice overuse, may resolve with vocal rest or therapy	Hoarseness, change in voice quality, difficulty speaking and singing, vocal fatigue, sore throat
		Vocal cord polyps: stalk-like growth, larger than nodules, usually unilateral	Symptoms similar to that of vocal cord nodules

Abbreviations: *CNS* central nervous system, *ET* endotracheal, *GERD* gastroesophageal reflux disease, *HPV* human papillomavirus, *MS* multiple sclerosis, *PND* postnasal drip, *SLE* systemic lupus erythematosus, *TB* tuberculosis, *UES* upper esophageal sphincter, *URI* upper respiratory infection

Pathophysiology in Allergic Rhinitis

Introduction to Allergic Rhinitis

AR is a common disorder associated with a symptom complex characterized primarily by nasal but associated with non-nasal symptoms. Individuals with the conditions usually experience sneezing, anterior and posterior rhinorrhea, nasal congestion, itching of the eyes, nose, and palate, as well as PND and cough. The disease is termed allergic rhinoconjunctivitis if ocular symptoms are present (Bousquet et al. 2020). AR usually presents in childhood and adolescence, with most affected individuals developing symptoms before the age of 20 years and roughly half of these patients before the age of 6 years. AR frequently presents with atopic eczema and asthma in early childhood as part of an inherited syndrome (atopy).

Risk factors for AR include family history of allergic diseases, male sex in children, firstborn status, birth during a major pollen season, maternal smoking, indoor allergen exposure, and early-life antibiotic use (Schuler IV & Montejo 2019). Symptoms and severity are influenced by age and allergen exposure. Children with AR tend to have symptoms that are more intermittent (last $\leq$4 days a week or $\leq$ 4 weeks), moderate/severe classification (based on the presence or absence of sleep disturbance, impairment of daily activities including school, work, leisure and or sports), and associated with high frequency of comorbidities (asthma, conjunctivitis, and atopic dermatitis). Adults tend to have perennial AR, while children and adolescents suffer more frequently from seasonal AR (Izquierdo-Domínguez et al. 2017). This condition significantly affects quality of life by contributing to fatigue, depression, sleep disruption, and impaired attention, learning, and memory (Schuler IV & Montejo 2019).

Antigen Sensitization and Re-exposure

AR begins with a sensitization phase driven by allergen exposure and deposition onto the nasal mucosa. Airborne allergens include pollens (from grasses, weeds, and trees), fungal spores and other fungal products, and animal allergens. APCs in the submucosa and lymphoid tissue process the antigens and present peptide fragments on class II major histocompatibility complex molecules to naïve CD4+ T cells (Nur Husna et al. 2022). Type 2 inflammation is activated and is characterized by overexpression and increased release of cytokines, histamine, and other mediators. Nasal epithelial barrier damage or irritation from allergic inflammation or irritants (e.g. pollutants, combustion products, viral infection) triggers the release of alarmins (IL-25, IL-33, thymic stromal lymphopoietin from epithelial cells, which contribute to the type 2 inflammation. Some allergens, such as dust mite allergens, accentuate epithelial damage further with proteases. The epithelial alarmins recruit granulocytes (eosinophils and basophils) and activate mast cells, dendritic cells, and type 2 innate lymphoid cells (ILC2s). Activated ILC2s produce IL-4, IL-5, IL-13, and IL-31.

While the type 2 inflammatory response typically leads to epithelial damage with a barrier repair response, allergic conditions with continuous or recurrent barrier compromise may result in chronic inflammation that overcomes the repair processes. Type 2 inflammation also drives neuroimmune activation with sensitization of mucosal sensory neurons to non-specific irritants and other stimuli. The clinical implications of neuroimmune activity vary by tissue type and disease state (Bousquet et al. 2020). Persistent, severe type 2 inflammatory response, related to allergy or non-allergic disease, may result in the development of CRSwNP. Nasal polyp mucosal tissue contains an increased number of T cells, eosinophils, basophils, and mast cells and high levels of IL-4, IL-5, IL-13, and IgE (type 2 polarization), which lead to hypersecretion of mucus and decrease olfactory function (Helman et al. 2020).

Isotype switching to IgE results from the rearrangement of germline DNA in the C (constant domain)-epsilon locus of the Ig heavy chain in naïve B cells stimulated by IL-4 and IL-13 and the interaction between the B cell membrane-bound CD40 with the CD40 ligand on the surface of T lymphocytes. The presence of IL-4 and

IL-13 upregulates vascular cell-adhesion molecule 1 on endothelial cells, resulting in the migration of inflammatory cells, particularly eosinophils, into areas of allergic inflammation (Nur Husna et al. 2022). After exposure to allergens, the allergic nasal mucosa has increased amounts of mRNA expressing IL-3, IL-4, IL-5, IL-13, eotaxins (selective chemoattractants for eosinophils), and granulocyte-macrophage colony-stimulating factor (GM-CSF) and a reduction of interferon-gamma, IL-12, and IL-18 (Nur Husna et al. 2022; Bjermer et al. 2019).

Allergen-specific IgE (sIgE) binds to high-affinity Fc-epsilon receptors on the respiratory mucosa's effector cells (mast cells and basophils) and enhances type 2 inflammation following repeat allergen exposure. Upon re-encountering the causative antigen, sIgE crosslinks on mast cells and initiates a type I hypersensitivity reaction involving mast cell activation and release of granule-associated chemical mediators and stimulation of production of other mediators. Memory B cells and long-lived plasma cells are responsible for maintaining the production of sIgE.

In AR, Th2 cytokines activate mucosal mast cells to proliferate and result in an increase in the number of mast cells and basophils in the superficial nasal epithelium compared with subjects without AR. Th2 cytokines further propagate inflammation by disrupting the sinonasal epithelial cell barrier, increasing mucosal permeability, and interfering with barrier repair, which increases mucosal susceptibility to irritants and infections and augments response to repeat nasal allergen exposure (nasal priming) (Bousquet et al. 2020).

Downstream Mediators of Allergic Inflammation and URT Mucosal Injury

Chemical mediators released or formed during mast cell degranulation include histamine, prostaglandins (PGDs), leukotrienes (LTs), platelet-activating factor (PAF), proteases, and bradykinin (Bousquet et al. 2020; Bjermer et al. 2019). The release of preformed histamine from mast cells interacts with H1 and H2 receptors on postcapillary venules and H1 receptors on sensory nerve fibers, propagating inflammation through vasodilation, increased vascular permeability, and stimulation of sensory nerve fibers. All of these contribute to the clinically observed symptoms of AR, including nasal congestion, rhinorrhea, mucosal edema, pruritus, and sneezing (sneeze reflex).

Phospholipase A2 is involved in mast cell activation by stimulating the release of arachidonic acid from cell membrane lipids. Arachidonic acid is then metabolized by either the cyclooxygenase pathway forming PGD2 and thromboxane mediators or the lipoxygenase pathway forming LTC4, LTD4, and LTE4. Notably, PGD2 is a more potent stimulator of nasal congestion than histamine (Nur Husna et al. 2022; Bjermer et al. 2019).

The inflammatory reaction in AR is also amplified by the release of cytokines from mast cells, including GM-CSF, tumor necrosis factor (TNF) alpha, transforming growth factor beta, IL-1, IL-4, IL-5, IL-6, IL-9, and IL-13. These mediators promote further IgE production, eosinophil and mast cell growth or activation, inflammatory cell chemotaxis, and enhanced eosinophil and possibly mast cell survival. In tissue from individuals with AR, eosinophilia results from the IL-5, TNF-alpha, and IL-1-mediated expression of eosinophil adhesion receptors on the endothelium. Furthermore, eosinophils promote Th2 cell proliferation and mast cell growth by releasing multiple cytokines, including IL-3, IL-4, IL-5, IL-10, and GM-CSF. Of these cytokines, IL-3, IL-5, and GM-CSF additionally potentiate hematopoiesis, differentiation, and survival of eosinophils. Thus, these interactions establish a perpetuation of the type 2 response (Bousquet et al. 2020; Bjermer et al. 2019).

Lastly, eosinophils contribute to nasal epithelial injury, desquamation, subepithelial fibrosis, and neural hyperresponsiveness via the release of oxygen radicals and proteins such as eosinophil major basic protein, eosinophil peroxidases, eosinophil neurotoxin, and eosinophil cationic protein. Therefore, in an allergic response, the activation of eosinophils and mast cells leads to the expression of adhesion molecules on vascular endothelial cells, followed by the vascular endothelial adhesion of leukocytes, transendothelial migration, and persistent inflammation.

Chemokines such as RANTES (regulated on activation, normal T cell expressed and secreted), eotaxins, and monocyte chemotactic proteins 3 and 4 also enhance the migration and activation of inflammatory cells in the nasal mucosa during allergic reactions. In AR, nitric oxide production in the nasal mucosa by mast cells, neutrophils, endothelial, and epithelial cells causes vasodilation and nasal obstruction. This physiology similarly affects the sinus mucosa, predisposing to CRS (Nur Husna et al. 2022; Bousquet et al. 2020).

Early and Late Phase Reactions

The type 1 allergic response in general and AR in particular is divided into two phases: early (immediate) and late (hours later). The early phase begins within seconds to minutes of allergen exposure and peaks at 15–30 min. It is characterized by mast cell degranulation in the nasal mucosa, releasing preformed granule mediators, including histamine and newly synthesized mediators. Additionally, large quantities of type 2 cytokines such as IL-4, IL-5, and IL-13 are produced by PGD2-recruited and activated ILC2s; even several hours after allergen exposure, these cytokines can be detected in nasal tissue and secretions. Histamine and PGD2 levels return to baseline after approximately 30 min.

The late phase reaction peaks around 6–12 h after allergen exposure. Chronic AR is related to this secondary inflammatory response and the second release of mediators. Roughly 3–11 h after allergen exposure, cytokines IL-4 and IL-5 trigger the influx of T-cells, basophils, neutrophils, monocytes, and eosinophils into the nasal mucosa. All the early-phase mediators contribute to the late phase based on nasal challenge models except for PGD2; PGD2 is not produced by basophils, suggesting that these are one of the primary cell mediators in this phase.

Lymphocytes are found in the nasal mucosa following allergen exposure. These cells have increased expression of the IL-2 receptor and participate in transcription for IL-3, IL-4, IL-5, and GM-CSF (Nur Husna et al. 2022; Bjermer et al. 2019). Two other phenomena have been noted in AR: nasal priming and nasal hyper-responsiveness to non-allergen stimuli (see above). Nasal priming refers to low pollen counts (lower than required for initial symptom induction) triggering AR symptoms during the waning pollen season. In this phenomenon, repeat allergen exposure causes an increased accumulation of mast cells and basophils in the nasal mucosa at the site of the allergic reaction (Bousquet et al. 2020).

Nasal Allergen Provocation Testing and Nasal Sampling

Nasal allergen provocation testing (NAPT) can be helpful in the diagnosis of seasonal and perennial AR, occupational rhinitis, and local allergic rhinitis (LAR). This diagnostic tool is primarily utilized in asymptomatic or mildly symptomatic patients. A single allergen is applied to the nasal mucosa, followed by nasal sampling through techniques like brushing/scraping, bulk and focal surface fluid collection, and turbinate biopsy to evaluate for mucosal inflammation. These objective assays are combined with symptom scores to assess the challenge results (Bousquet et al. 2020).

Each nasal sampling technique has advantages and challenges. Nasal brushing is fast, does not require topical anesthesia or endoscopic guidance, and may yield more cells than nasal lavage; however, the ability to collect inflammatory mediators is inconsistent, and vigorous brushing may lead to patient discomfort and poor sample yield. Nasal aspiration and nasal lavage are both fast, inexpensive, and do not require topical anesthesia. Challenges with nasal aspiration include the difficulty in assessing for dilution factor and blind suctioning-induced nasal mucosal trauma. The difficulties with nasal lavage include patient compliance, overly diluted samples, variability in the path of lavage fluid flow, and inability to isolate fluid from specific regions. Mucosal biopsy allows for histologic evaluation, though topical anesthesia is often required, the technique is more time-consuming, trauma is involved with patient discomfort and the risk of epistaxis, and serial exams are usually not feasible. Such techniques are used in research protocols and may be used clinically to diagnose LAR (see below) (Massey et al. 2020).

Local Allergic Rhinitis

LAR is a unique form of AR with clinical symptoms similar to AR; however, systemic atopy as identified by specific-IgE in enzyme-linked assays of the blood or positive allergen skin tests is absent. The primary feature of LAR is a T and B cell-driven allergic response that is limited to the nasal mucosa and lacks peripheral specific-IgE. This local response results in a positive NAPT but negative allergen skin testing and in vitro testing (Campo & Canonica 2024).

Neurophysiology of Allergic Rhinitis

The nasal physiology in AR is affected by the decreased sympathetic tone and increased cholinergic tone, resulting in arterial dilation and engorgement of the sinusoidal erectile tissue, as well as passive diffusion of plasma proteins into the URT and increased mucus gland cell secretion. Additionally, after allergen exposure in AR, nasal secretions containing neurotransmitters such as substance P, CGRP, and VIP, contribute to neurogenic stimulation and increased local blood flow and glandular secretion. Mucosal inflammation can persistently upregulate neural function. Sensory neural stimulation may result in antidromic stimulation (a spreading of stimulus along the multiple branches of a sensory neuron) of nociceptive sensory fibers. This neural stimulation releases tachykinins (i.e., substance P and neurokinin A) and CGRP, causing an increase in neurogenic inflammation (Baroody 2007).

Olfaction is an important neural function of the URT. Hyposmia affects roughly 23% of individuals with AR and is primarily a result of nasal passage obstruction and inflammation in the olfactory cleft. Research using validated questionaries shows that hyposmia significantly impacts AR patients' quality of life. Conversely, quality of life improves in AR patients with improved olfaction post-therapy of AR (Stuck & Hummel 2015). Hyposmia is more prevalent in individuals with sinus disease such as CRSwNP, where olfactory dysfunction is observed in roughly 90%. Similar to AR, improved olfaction among patients with CRSwNP results in an enhanced quality of life (Helman et al. 2020).

Summary and Conclusion

In conclusion, the URT is the first line of defense against respiratory pathogens through innate, adaptive, and acquired immunity, as well as neurosensory responses. Understanding the anatomy and pathophysiology of the URT provides a framework for appreciating the immunologic mechanisms in AR and the explanation for symptoms. Knowledge of the URT anatomy also facilitates the differential diagnosis by assisting in the recognition of conditions other than AR that are responsible for symptoms. The early and late phases of AR highlight the importance of APCs, sIgE, and activation of Th2 cells, B cells, eosinophils, basophils, and mast cells, resulting in variable release of multiple mediators and the clinical manifestations of sneezing, rhinorrhea, nasal congestion, and itching.

Additionally, AR contributes to fatigue, depression, sleep disturbance, hyposmia, and impaired cognition, significantly impairing the quality of life in affected subjects. Understanding both the anatomy and pathophysiology of AR will potentially lead to improved diagnosis and possibly novel therapies for this common condition. Ultimately, the interpretation of this complex pathophysiology of AR is predicated on an understanding and awareness of the anatomy, physiology, and immunity of the URT.FundingThis research did not receive any specific grant from funding agencies in the public, commercial, or not-for-profit sectors.

References

Anniko M, Bernal-Sprekelsen M, et al. European manual of medicine – otorhinolaryngology, head and neck surgery. Surgery. 2010:140.

Baroody FM. Nasal and paranasal sinus anatomy and physiology. Clin Allergy Immunol. 2007;19:1–21.

Belafsky PC, Lintzenich CR. Development, anatomy, and physiology of the pharynx. In: Principles of deglutition: a multidisciplinary text for swallowing and its disorders. Springer New York; 2013.

Bjermer L, Westman M, Holmström M, Wickman MC. The complex pathophysiology of allergic rhinitis: scientific rationale for the development of an alternative treatment option. Allergy Asthma Clin Immunol. 2019;15

Bousquet J, Anto JM, Bachert C, Baiardini I, Bosnic-Anticevich S, Walter Canonica G, et al. Allergic rhinitis. Nat Rev Dis Prim. 2020;6(1):95.

Campo P, Canonica GW. Local allergic rhinitis. J Allergy Clin Immunol Pract. 2024;12(6):1430–3.

Di Cicco M, Kantar A, Masini B, Nuzzi G, Ragazzo V, Peroni D. Structural and functional development in airways throughout childhood: Children are not small adults. Pediatr Pulmonol. 2021;56(1):240–51.

Helman SN, Barrow E, Edwards T, DelGaudio JM, Levy JM, Wise SK. The role of allergic rhinitis in chronic rhinosinusitis. Immunol Allergy Clin N Am. 2020;40:201–14.

Izquierdo-Domínguez A, Jauregui I, del Cuvillo A, Montoro J, Dávila I, Sastre J, et al. Allergy rhinitis: similarities and differences between children and adults. Rhinology. 2017;55(4):326–31.

Lee S, Fernandez J, Mirjalili SA, Kirkpatrick J. Pediatric paranasal sinuses – development, growth, pathology, & functional endoscopic sinus surgery. Clin Anat. 2022;35

Marcus S, Schertzer J, Roland LT, Wise SK, Levy JM, DelGaudio JM. Central compartment atopic disease: prevalence of allergy and asthma compared with other subtypes of chronic rhinosinusitis with nasal polyps. Int Forum Allergy Rhinol. 2020;10(2):183–9.

Massey CJ, Diaz Del Valle F, Abuzeid WM, Levy JM, Mueller S, Levine CG, et al. Sample collection for laboratory-based study of the nasal airway and sinuses: a research compendium. Int Forum Allergy Rhinol. 2020;10(3):303–13.

Neskey D, Eloy JA, Casiano RR. Nasal, septal, and turbinate anatomy and embryology. Otolaryngol Clin N Am. 2009;42:193–205.

Nur Husna SM, Tan HTT, Md Shukri N, Mohd Ashari NS, Wong KK. Allergic rhinitis: a clinical and pathophysiological overview. Front Med. 2022;9

Önerci TM. Nasal physiology and pathophysiology of nasal disorders. In: Nasal physiology and pathophysiology of nasal disorders. Springer Berlin Heidelberg; 2013.

Pedan H, Janosova V, Hajtman A, Calkovsky V. Non-reflex defense mechanisms of upper airway mucosa: possible clinical application. Physiol Res. 2020;69:S55–67.

Sahin-Yilmaz A, Naclerio RM. Anatomy and physiology of the upper airway. Ann Am Thorac Soc. 2011;8:31–9.

Schuler CF IV, Montejo JM. Allergic rhinitis in children and adolescents. Pediatr Clin N Am. 2019;66:981–93.

Smallwood D, Ledford D, Kennedy D, Lockey R. Postnasal drip. J Allergy Clin Immunol Pract. 2024;12(6):1472–8.

Stuck BA, Hummel T. Olfaction in allergic rhinitis: a systematic review. J Allergy Clin Immunol. 2015;136:1460–70.

Trachsel D, et al. Developmental respiratory physiology. Paediatr Anaesth. 2022;32:108–17.

Chapter 2
Common Aeroallergens and Aerobiology of North America

Ann Printy, Zachary Hostoffer, Jack Jeskey, Nicole Tierney, Devi Jhaveri, and Robert W. Hostoffer

Introduction

The effects of aeroallergens were first described by Dr. John Bostock, M.D. in 1819. In his work, *A Case of the Periodical Affection of the Eyes and Chest*, he offered a detailed depiction of the ocular, nasal, and pulmonary symptoms he experienced during warmer weather. Later in 1828, he introduced the name "catarrhus aestivus" (Catarrhus meaning "to flow down" and aestivus meaning "summer") to describe the recurrent sneezing, nasal drainage, and congestion he experienced and attributed to heat exposure. These symptoms were later called "hay fever," as symptoms seemed to be pronounced during hay harvesting in the spring and summer. In 1873, Dr. Charles Blackley conducted a series of experiments on himself as well as airborne pollen to identify the true culprit of pollinosis. By 1906, Von Pirquet introduced the concept of an "allergen" to describe a particle that was able to trigger an immune reaction, and by the 1920s the notion of "atopy" or that certain individuals had increased odds of becoming sensitized had emerged. By the 1980s, research identified numerous IgE-mediated allergens. There are currently 1095 allergens which have been identified, and nearly 50% are airborne. Allergic rhinitis is becoming increasingly prevalent, with symptoms affecting patients at younger ages. In the

A. Printy
Department of Medical Education, Pediatric Residency Program, Akron Children's Hospital, Akron, OH, USA

Z. Hostoffer
St John Internal Medicine Residency, University Hospitals, Westlake, OH, USA

J. Jeskey · D. Jhaveri · R. W. Hostoffer (✉)
Cleveland Medical Center, University Hospitals, Cleveland, OH, USA

N. Tierney
University of Northern Iowa, Cedar Falls, IA, USA

M. Mahmoudi (ed.), *Treatment and Management of Allergic Rhinitis*,
https://doi.org/10.1007/978-3-031-88107-7_2

United States, an estimated 50 million people are diagnosed with allergic rhinitis, with 40% developing symptoms before age six and 80% developing by age 20. The cost of care for allergic rhinitis is estimated to be $3.4 billion annually, and with the added burden of missed work and school due to symptoms, it is no surprise that it has become a significant public health concern.

General Principles of Allergen Aerobiology

Aerobiology is the study of airborne particles that originate from, or are a byproduct of, living organisms. The field examines the factors which influence production, distribution, and prevalence of these particles. Common airborne allergens include pollen grains, fungal spores, insect feces, and animal dander. Aeroallergens can be described by their chemical composition, stability, and solubility, which all determine the bioavailability of the compound. Additionally, these allergens can be categorized into outdoor or indoor particles and can be seasonal or perennial. Outdoor aeroallergens such as fungal spores and pollen, are affected by external factors such as humidity, precipitation, temperature, ultraviolet radiation, and air quality. Indoor aeroallergens also include fungal spores, as well as compounds from animals and insects. Similarly, they are impacted by humidity, ventilation, and building materials. These factors may individually alter the availability of aeroallergens; however, it is important to acknowledge how they will operate in consortium to generate overall amplification or reduction. Aeroallergens are not intrinsically pathogenic but when transmitted to the nasal passages of a susceptible individual they can elicit an immune response. Upon initial exposure, certain individuals will become sensitized and produce allergen-specific IgE antibodies. Following repeated exposure, the aerosol binds to specific IgE antibodies located on mast cells and basophils, which leads to activation and release of inflammatory mediators (histamine, prostaglandins, leukotrienes, cytokines), inducing the symptoms of rhinitis. With the immune response to allergens in mind, it is essential to investigate how aeroallergens are produced, distributed, and respond to environmental change.

Production and Release of Aeroallergens

Allergen producing organisms have individual ideal environmental conditions, however, identifying general patterns is important for disease epidemiology. Pollen is produced during the reproductive cycle of plants, including trees, grasses, and weeds. Pollen calendars are helpful as the timing of pollen release and mechanisms of dispersal are variable and plant specific. Some plants require vernalization or changes in photoperiod for pollen to be produced, and generally earlier start dates are seen at lower latitudes in North America. Fungi rely on organic matter in the environment for their growth and reproduction. In a manner like flowering plants, fungi propagate by releasing spores, which are also recognized to contain allergenic components. In northern latitudes, outdoor fungal spores increase in spring until peaking in early fall, while in southern latitudes levels are nearly continuous and are limited by humidity and high temperature. Other common sources of allergens originate from insects and animals and can be found in indoor environments. Insects such as mites and cockroaches create allergens through their body fragments and feces. Household pets produce allergens through dander, saliva, and excrement. To promote primary prevention, it is important to recognize where these particles originate from and how they traverse the environment to arrive in the respiratory tract of humans.

Dispersion and Transport

Aeroallergens can be dispersed through either passive or active mechanisms. They may be carried through the air by passive wind, either natural or mechanical, or through active dispersal during fungal discharge. Once airborne, the movement of particles can be influenced by wind speed, turbulence, and vertical mixing, which may determine their dispersion over land. For instance, certain grass pollen can travel hundreds of miles under appropriate wind direction as opposed to heavier particles, such as fungal spores, which tend to settle more quickly. Weather conditions, such as precipitation and air pressure, impact aeroallergen concentration. In the case of pollen, rainfall helps decrease allergens from the air, while thunderstorms crack pollen grains into smaller fragments, which facilitates entrance into the respiratory tract.

Persistence and Environmental Interactions

The timing and intensity of allergen release depend on environmental factors such as temperature, humidity, and light, as well as the life cycles of the producing organisms.

Smaller particles may be sustained in the environment for longer periods of time and enter the respiratory tract more easily. The stability of these aeroallergens may also be affected by ultraviolet radiation, moisture, and microbial degradation. Indoor environments, characterized by reduced air exchange and stable temperatures, often promote accumulation of allergens such as dust mites and pet dander. These persistent particles can contribute to overall increases in allergen concentration and exposure, negatively impacting susceptible individuals.

Host Interaction and Sensitization

The human biological potency of aeroallergens is a function of their ability to bind to IgE antibodies and trigger immune responses. Particle size plays a critical role in determining allergen deposition within the respiratory tract, with larger particles >10 mm primarily affecting the upper airways and smaller particles <5 mm reaching the lower airways. Increased allergenicity is associated with daily sequential exposure. Additionally, allergen structure, including protein composition and enzymatic activity, can influence allergenicity. For example, certain allergens possess proteolytic enzymes that disrupt epithelial barriers and enhance immune sensitization. One way this may occur is through the stimulation of protease activated receptors, which are G-protein coupled receptors which can release chemokines, cytokines, and metalloproteinases upon activation. Protease activated receptors have also been linked to increased IgE production, smooth muscle hypertrophy, and fibroblast proliferation.

Temporal and Geographic Variability

Aeroallergen levels exhibit significant temporal and geographic variability. Seasonal fluctuations in pollen and fungal spore concentrations are well-documented, reflecting the reproductive cycles of plants and fungi. Geographic factors, such as vegetation type, urbanization, and climate, also shape allergen profiles in different regions. Urban areas, for example, may experience higher exposure to certain indoor allergens due to confined living conditions, while rural areas may encounter elevated levels of outdoor allergens like pollen. By integrating knowledge of allergen production, dispersion, and host interaction, allergen aerobiology provides a foundation for developing strategies to reduce exposure and manage allergic diseases. Advances in aerobiological monitoring and modeling also hold promise for improving predictive capabilities and informing public health interventions.

Characterized Allergens

Allergens are specific proteins or glycoproteins that elicit IgE-mediated immune responses in sensitized individuals. These biologically active molecules are derived from a wide range of sources, including plants, fungi, arthropods, and animals. Characterizing allergens involves understanding their origin, molecular properties, and biological functions, all of which are crucial for developing diagnostic tools, immunotherapy treatments, and strategies to mitigate allergen exposure.

Plant-Derived Allergens

Pollen is a major source of plant allergens, particularly from grasses, trees, and weeds. These allergens are typically small, soluble proteins that can easily cross mucosal barriers in the respiratory tract. For example, Bet v 1, the major birch pollen allergen, is a pathogenesis-related protein involved in plant defense mechanisms. Grass pollens, such as Lol p 1 from ryegrass, are highly allergenic due to their abundance and widespread distribution. Weed pollens, such as Amb a 1 from ragweed, are notable for their ability to cause severe allergic reactions and widespread sensitization.

Fungal Allergens

Fungi are another significant source of airborne allergens, primarily in the form of spores and hyphal fragments. Common fungal allergens include those from *Alternaria alternata* (Alt a 1) and *Cladosporium herbarum* (Cla h 1). These proteins are often enzymes, such as proteases and glycoside hydrolases, that facilitate fungal growth and interaction with host tissues. The allergenic potential of fungi is enhanced by their ability to grow in diverse environments and produce high concentrations of airborne spores, particularly in damp indoor settings and during specific seasons.

Arthropod-Derived Allergens

Dust mites and cockroaches are key arthropod sources of allergens. Dust mite allergens, such as Der p 1 and Der f 1, are proteolytic enzymes found in mite feces. These allergens are particularly potent due to their ability to disrupt epithelial barriers and stimulate robust immune responses. Cockroach allergens, such as Bla g 1 and Bla g 2, are associated with asthma and allergic rhinitis, especially in urban environments with poor sanitation. These allergens are often carried on small particles, allowing them to remain airborne and penetrate deep into the respiratory tract.

Animal-Derived Allergens

Animal allergens are commonly found in dander, saliva, and urine from pets such as cats and dogs. Fel d 1, the major cat allergen, is a secretoglobin produced in the sebaceous and salivary glands. Dog allergens, such as Can f 1 and Can f 5, are lipocalins that serve various biological roles, including pheromone transport. Rodents, such as mice and rats, also produce allergens that are significant occupational hazards in laboratory and agricultural settings. Animal allergens are highly adhesive and can persist in indoor environments, making them difficult to eliminate entirely.

Cross-reactivity and Molecular Homology

Many allergens exhibit cross-reactivity due to molecular homology, where structurally similar proteins from different sources elicit similar immune responses. For instance, Bet v 1 from birch pollen is homologous to certain food allergens, leading to oral allergy syndrome in individuals sensitized to birch. Similarly, tropomyosins, a class of muscle proteins, are shared across arthropods such as dust mites, shellfish, and cockroaches, contributing to cross-reactivity between these allergen sources. Understanding these relationships is essential for accurate diagnosis and personalized allergen avoidance strategies. The characterization of allergens at the molecular level provides valuable insights into their immunogenicity, stability, and environmental persistence. This knowledge underpins advancements in allergen-specific immunotherapy and the development of hypoallergenic variants for treatment. By elucidating the structural and functional properties of allergens, researchers can enhance their ability to manage allergic diseases and improve patient outcomes.

Aeroallergen Sampling

The accurate identification and quantification of aeroallergens are critical for understanding exposure levels, assessing health risks, and developing mitigation strategies. Various sampling techniques have been developed to capture and analyze airborne allergens, each tailored to specific study objectives, environmental conditions, and allergen types. These methods can be broadly categorized into passive and active sampling, with each having distinct advantages and limitations.

Passive Sampling

Passive samplers rely on the natural settling of airborne particles onto collection surfaces. Common passive sampling devices include adhesive-coated slides, sticky tapes, and settling plates. These methods are simple, cost-effective, and do not require specialized equipment, making them ideal for long-term environmental monitoring. However, passive samplers provide limited temporal resolution and are influenced by environmental factors such as wind speed and gravity. While useful for qualitative assessments, passive sampling is less effective for quantifying allergen concentrations or capturing particles with low sedimentation rates.

Active Sampling

Active sampling techniques involve the use of mechanical devices to draw air through a collection medium, such as filters, impaction surfaces, or liquid impingers. These methods provide precise control over sampling volumes and durations, enabling quantitative measurements of allergen concentrations.

Impaction Samplers: Devices such as the Rotorod Sampler, Burkard or Hirst volumetric samplers collect airborne particles onto adhesive-coated surfaces by directing airflow against a solid impactor. These samplers are widely used for pollen and fungal spore monitoring due to their ability to capture a broad size range of particles and provide high temporal resolution.

Filter-Based Samplers: High-volume air samplers draw air through filters made of materials like glass fiber or polycarbonate, which trap airborne particles for subsequent analysis. These samplers are versatile and suitable for collecting a wide range of aeroallergens, including pollen, fungal spores, and particulate-bound allergens like dust mite feces and pet dander.

Liquid Impingers: In these devices, air is bubbled through a liquid medium, such as saline or buffer solution, which captures aerosolized particles. Liquid impingers are particularly effective for sampling allergenic proteins and bioaerosols, as the captured particles remain suspended in solution, facilitating downstream biochemical and immunological analyses.

Analysis and Quantification

After collection, aeroallergens are analyzed using techniques such as microscopy, immunoassays, and molecular methods. Light and electron microscopy are commonly employed for identifying pollen and fungal spores based on morphological characteristics. Enzyme-linked immunosorbent assays (ELISA) and radioallergosorbent tests (RAST) are used to detect and quantify allergenic proteins. Molecular methods, including polymerase chain reaction (PCR) and next-generation sequencing (NGS), enable the identification of allergen genes and provide detailed insights into allergen diversity and abundance.

Integrated Sampling Approaches

Recent advances in aeroallergen sampling involve integrated systems that combine collection and analysis into a single platform. For example, real-time aerosol monitoring devices equipped with optical sensors can detect changes in airborne particle concentrations and composition, providing immediate data on allergen exposure. Additionally, automated samplers linked to meteorological sensors allow researchers to correlate allergen levels with environmental variables, such as temperature, humidity, and wind speed.

Challenges and Considerations

Despite their utility, aeroallergen sampling techniques face challenges related to variability in particle size, distribution, and environmental conditions. The selection of an appropriate sampling method depends on the target allergen, study objectives, and resource availability. For instance, while impaction samplers are excellent for capturing large pollen grains, they may under-sample smaller particles such as fungal spores or allergenic proteins. Furthermore, preserving the integrity of collected allergens during transport and storage is essential for accurate analysis.

The ongoing development of advanced sampling and analytical techniques continues to enhance the field of aeroallergen monitoring. These innovations hold promise for improving allergen exposure assessments, enabling more precise predictions of allergic disease trends, and informing public health interventions.

Representative Pollens

Pollen is a significant aeroallergen in the United States, contributing to seasonal allergic rhinitis, commonly known as hay fever, and other allergic conditions. The main sources of allergenic pollen are trees, grasses, and weeds, with each group exhibiting distinct seasonal and geographic patterns. Understanding the diversity of pollen types and their distribution is essential for managing pollen-related allergies and forecasting exposure risks.

Tree Pollen

Tree pollen is a major contributor to springtime allergies in the United States. Common allergenic trees include birch (*Betula*), oak (*Quercus*), cedar (*Juniperus*), maple (*Acer*), and elm (Ulmus)) (Table 2.1). These trees release large quantities of pollen during their reproductive cycles, typically from late winter to early summer,

Table 2.1 Major tree pollens in North America

Order	Family	Genus and species	Common name
Pinales	Cupressaceae	*Chamaecyparis obtusa*	Hinoki cypress
		Hesperocyparis arizonica	Arizona cypress
		Cupressus sempervirens	Mediterranean cypress
		Cryptomeria japonica	Japanese cedar
		Juniperus ashei	Mountain cedar
		Juniperus virginiana	Red cedar
		Juniperus oxycedrus	Prickly juniper
		Juniperus communis	Common juniper
Arecales	Arecaceae	*Phoenix dactylifera*	Date palm
Proteales	Platanaceae	*Platanus* × *acerifolia* (hybrid species)	London plane tree
		Platanus orientalis	Oriental plane tree
		Platanus occidentalis	American sycamore
		Platanus racemosa	California sycamore
		Platanus wrightii	Arizona sycamore

(continued)

Table 2.1 (continued)

Order	Family	Genus and species	Common name
Laminales	Oleaceae	*Ligustrum vulgare*	Common privet
		Olea europaea	Olive tree
		Syringa vulgaris	Common lilac
		Fraxinus excelsior	Common ash
		Fraxinus americana	White ash
		Fraxinus pennsylvanica	Green ash
		Fraxinus latifolia	Oregon ash
Fabales	Fabaceae	*Prosopis juliflora*	Mesquite tree
		Peltophorum pterocarpum	Yellow Peltophorum
Fagales	Fagaceae	*Castanea sativa*	European chestnut
		Fagus sylvatica	Common beech
		Quercus alba	White oak
		Quercus rubra	Red oak
		Quercus garryana	Oregon white oak
		Quercus gambelii	Gambel's oak
	Betulaceae	*Ostrya carpinifolia*	Hornbeam hop tree
		Betula pendula	Silver birch
		Betula papyrifera	Paper birch
		Betula occidentalis	Water birch
		Corylus avellana	Common hazel
		Corylus americana	American hazelnut
		Carpinus betulus	European hornbeam
		Carpinus caroliniana	American hornbeam
		Alnus glutinosa	Black alder
		Alnus incana rugosa	Speckled alder
		Alnus rubra	Red alder
	Juglandaceae	*Juglans nigra*	Black walnut
		Juglans californica	California walnut
		Juglans major	Arizona walnut
		Carya illinoinensis	Pecan
Sapindales	Sapindaceae	*Acer rubrum*	Red maple
		Acer saccharum	Sugar maple
		Acer negundo	Boxelder
		Acer macrophyllum	Big-leaved maple
Rosales	Ulmaceae	*Ulmus americana*	American elm
		Ulmus pumila	Siberian elm
		Ulmus parvifolia	Chinese elm
	Cannabaceae	*Celtis occidentalis*	Common hackberry
		Celtis ehrenbergiana	Torrey desert hackberry
	Moraceae	*Morus rubra*	Red mulberry
		Morus microphylla	Texas mulberry
Saxifragales	Altingiaceae	*Liquidambar styraciflua*	American sweetgum
Malpighiales	Salicaceae	*Salix nigra*	Black willow
		Populus alba	White poplar
		Populus sargentii	Western cottonwood

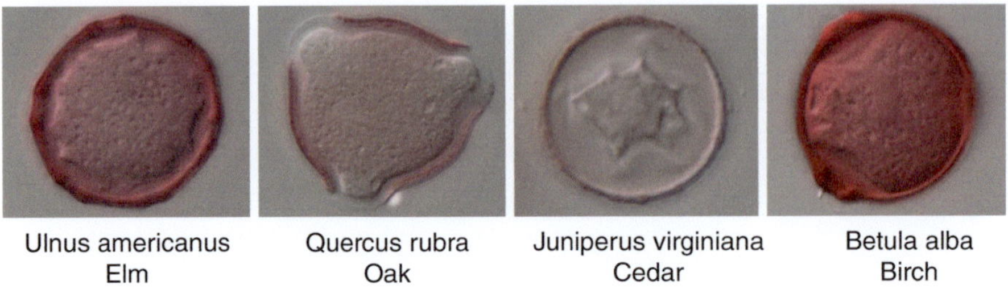

Fig. 2.1 Common tree pollens

Table 2.2 Major grass pollens in North America

Order and family	Subfamily	Genus and species	Common name
Poales Poaceae	Pooideae	*Lolium perenne*	Perennial ryegrass
		Festuca elatior	Meadow fescue
		Poa pratensis	Kentucky bluegrass
		Dactylis glomerata	Orchard grass
		Secale cereale	Rye
		Anthoxanthum odoratum	Sweet vernal grass
		Triticum aestivum	Wheat
		Avena sativa	Oats
		Phleum pratense	Timothy grass
		Agrostis stolonifera	Creeping bentgrass
	Chloridoideae	*Cynodon dactylon*	Bermuda grass
		Bouteloua dactyloides	Buffalo grass
	Arundinoideae	*Cortaderia selloana*	Pampas grass
	Panicoideae	*Paspalum notatum*	Bahia grass
		Sorghum halepense	Johnson grass
	Oryzoideae	*Oryza sativa*	Rice

depending on the species and region. Birch and oak pollen are particularly potent allergens, known to cause severe allergic reactions in sensitized individuals (Fig. 2.1). In the southern United States, cedar pollen, especially from mountain cedar (*Juniperus ashei*), is a significant allergen during late winter, a phenomenon often referred to as "cedar fever."

Grass Pollen

Grass pollen is a predominant allergen during late spring and summer, with peak seasons varying by region and grass species. In the United States, the most allergenic grasses include Kentucky bluegrass (*Poa pratensis*), Timothy grass (*Phleum pratense*), Bermuda grass (*Cynodon dactylon*), and ryegrass (*Lolium perenne*). (Table 2.2) Grass pollen is a common cause of outdoor allergies due to its

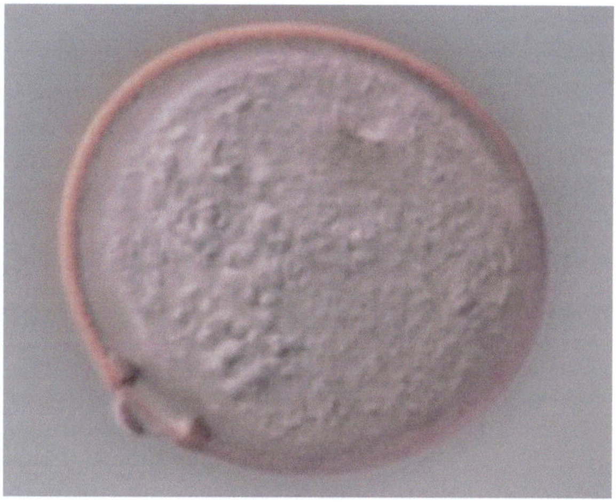

Fig. 2.2 Common grass pollen

widespread distribution and ability to travel long distances in the air. In the southeastern and western states, (Fig. 2.2) Bermuda grass is a notable allergen, while cool-season grasses like Kentucky bluegrass dominate in northern regions.

Weed Pollen

Weed pollen is a significant cause of fall allergies, with ragweed (*Ambrosia*) being the most notorious contributor. Ragweed pollen is highly allergenic and capable of traveling hundreds of miles, making it a widespread problem across much of the United States (Table 2.3, Fig. 2.3). Other allergenic weeds include sagebrush (*Artemisia)*, pigweed (*Amaranthus)*, lamb's quarters (*Chenopodium*), and Russian thistle (*Salsola*), commonly known as tumbleweed. These weeds thrive in disturbed soils and urban environments, contributing to high pollen levels in both rural and metropolitan areas.

Regional Variations

The diversity and concentration of pollen types vary significantly across the United States, influenced by climate, vegetation, and geography. For example, the northeastern states experience high levels of tree pollen in spring, followed by grass pollen in summer and ragweed pollen in fall. The southern states have a longer pollen season due to mild winters, with significant contributions from

Table 2.3 Major weed pollens in North America

Order	Family	Genus and species	Common name
Asterales	Asteraceae	*Ambrosia artemisiifolia*	Common ragweed
		Ambrosia elatior	Tall ragweed
		Ambrosia psilostachya	Western ragweed
		Ambrosia trifida	Giant ragweed
		Ambrosia bidentata	Two-toothed ragweed
		Ambrosia confertiflora	Desert ragweed
		Artemisia vulgaris	Mugwort
		Artemisia annua	Sweet wormwood
		Artemisia ludoviciana	Prairie sage
		Parthenium hysterophorus	Congress grass
		Helianthus annuus	Sunflower
		Chrysanthemum leucanthemum	Daisy
		Solidago gigantea	Goldenrod
		Taraxacum officinale	Dandelion
		Franseria acanthicarpa	False Goldenbush
		Franseria tenuifolia	Thinleaf Goldenbush
		Franseria ambrosioides	Ambrosia weed
		Xanthium communis	Common cocklebur
		Dicoria canescens	Gray Dicoria
Brassicales	Brassicaceae	*Brassica napus*	Rapeseed
		Brassica rapa	Turnip
Urticales	Urticaceae	*Parietaria judaica*	Wall Pellitory
		Parietaria officinalis	Common Pellitory
Malpighiales	Euphorbiaceae	*Mercurialis annua*	Annual mercury
Caryophyllales	Amaranthaceae	*Chenopodium album*	Lamb's quarters
		Salsola kali	Russian thistle
		Kochia scoparia	Burning bush
		Amaranthus retroflexus	Pigweed
	Polygonaceae	*Rumex acetosella*	Sheep Sorrel
		Rumex verticillatus	Swamp dock
		Rumex orbiculatus	Water dock
Lamiales	Plantaginaceae	*Plantago lanceolata*	English plantain
		Plantago rugelii	Blackseed Plaintain

tree, grass, and weed pollen throughout the year. In contrast, the arid southwestern states are characterized by high levels of weed pollen, including sagebrush and tumbleweed, while the Pacific Northwest has relatively low allergenic pollen levels due to its cooler, wetter climate and dominance of less allergenic vegetation like conifers.

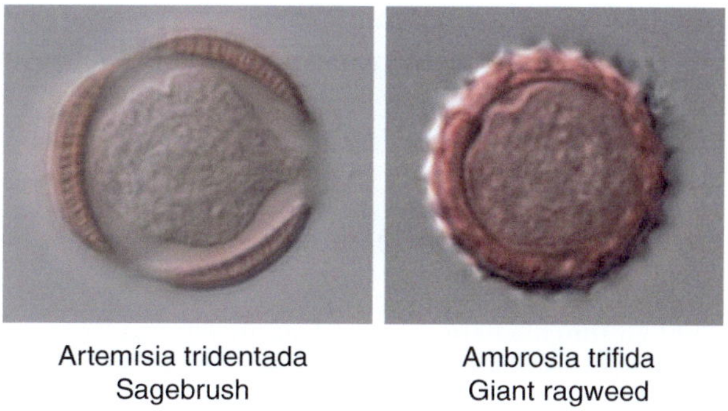

Fig. 2.3 Common weed pollens

Emerging Trends

Climate change is influencing the distribution, intensity, and seasonality of pollen in the United States. Warmer temperatures and increased atmospheric carbon dioxide levels are extending pollen seasons and enhancing pollen production for many allergenic plants, such as ragweed and grasses. Additionally, the introduction of non-native plant species and land-use changes are altering regional pollen profiles, potentially exposing populations to new allergens.

Efforts to monitor pollen levels and understand regional differences are essential for addressing the growing burden of pollen allergies in the United States. Advances in aerobiological research, predictive modeling, and public health initiatives can help mitigate the impact of allergenic pollen and improve the quality of life for affected individuals.

Pollen is a significant aeroallergen in the United States, contributing to seasonal allergic rhinitis (commonly known as hay fever) and other allergic conditions. The main sources of allergenic pollen are trees, grasses, and weeds, with each group exhibiting distinct seasonal and geographic patterns. Understanding the diversity of pollen types and their distribution is essential for managing pollen-related allergies and forecasting exposure risks.

Efforts to monitor pollen levels and understand regional differences are essential for addressing the growing burden of pollen allergies in the United States. Advances in aerobiological research, predictive modeling, and public health initiatives can help mitigate the impact of allergenic pollen and improve the quality of life for affected individuals.

Representative Fungi

Fungal aeroallergens are a significant contributor to allergic diseases such as allergic rhinitis, asthma, and hypersensitivity pneumonitis. In the United States, fungi release airborne spores and hyphal fragments that can trigger allergic reactions in sensitized individuals. These allergens are omnipresent in both indoor and outdoor environments, with their distribution influenced by climate, seasonality, and habitat.

Outdoor Fungal Allergens

Outdoor fungal allergens are primarily derived from molds that thrive in soil, decaying organic matter, and plant surfaces. The most allergenic outdoor fungi in the United States include *Alternaria, Cladosporium, Aspergillus*, and *Penicillium* (Table 2.4, Fig. 2.4).

Alternaria alternata is one of the most common fungal allergens, particularly in arid and temperate regions. Its spores are abundant during late summer and fall, often associated with the peak of the growing season. These small spores are highly aerodynamically efficient, allowing them to penetrate deep into the respiratory tract and trigger asthma and other allergic conditions.

Cladosporium species dominate outdoor fungal populations, especially during warm and humid conditions. These molds grow on plant surfaces and decaying leaves, releasing spores that are a common trigger of seasonal allergies.

Aspergillus and Penicillium are found in both outdoor and indoor environments. While typically associated with damp indoor conditions, these fungi can also be present in soil and decaying vegetation, releasing allergenic spores into the outdoor air.

Table 2.4 Common indoor and outdoor fungi

Class	Order	Family	Genus and species	Common name	Location
Dothideomycetes	Pleosporales	Pleosporaceae	*Alternaria alternata*	Alternaria	Primarily outdoor
	Cladosporiales	Cladosporiaceae	*Cladosporium herbarum*	Cladosporium	Primarily outdoor
Eurotiomycetes	Eurotiales	Trichocomaceae	*Penicillium Chrysogenum*	Penicillium	Indoor and outdoor
			Aspergillus fumigatus	Aspergillus	Indoor and outdoor
		Stachybotryaceae	*Stachybotrys chartarum*	Black mold	Indoor
Sordariomycetes	Sordariales	Chaetomiaceae	*Chaetomium globosum*	Chaetomium	Indoor

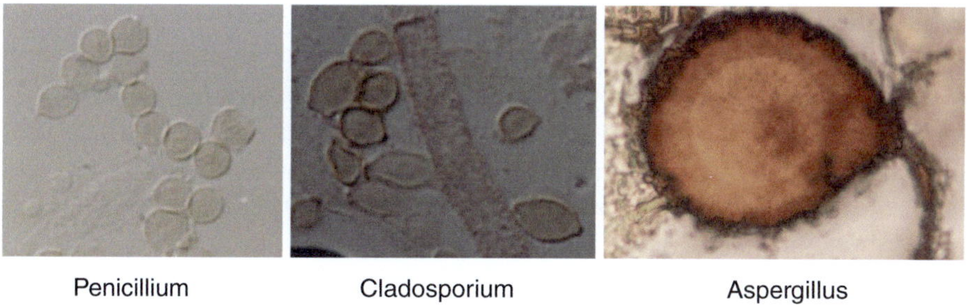

Fig. 2.4 Common fungus spores

Indoor Fungal Allergens

Indoor fungal allergens are predominantly associated with molds that thrive in damp or water-damaged environments. Key indoor allergenic fungi include *Aspergillus, Penicillium*, *Stachybotrys*, and *Chaetomium.*

Aspergillus fumigatus is a significant indoor allergen known for its role in allergic bronchopulmonary aspergillosis (ABPA) and hypersensitivity pneumonitis. It thrives in humid environments such as bathrooms, basements, and poorly ventilated spaces.

Penicillium species are highly diverse and commonly found indoors. Their spores are small and lightweight, allowing them to remain airborne for extended periods and infiltrate indoor air.

Stachybotrys chartarum, often referred to as "black mold," grows on water-damaged building materials such as drywall and wood. Although less common, its allergens and mycotoxins can cause severe respiratory and allergic reactions.

Chaetomium species are frequently associated with mold growth in damp indoor spaces. Their allergenic potential is often underestimated but poses risks to individuals with compromised immune systems or pre-existing allergies.

Seasonal and Regional Variations

The abundance and types of fungal aeroallergens vary seasonally and regionally in the United States. Outdoor fungal spores are most prevalent during warm and humid seasons, with peak concentrations in late summer and early fall. Regions with high humidity, such as the southeastern United States, experience elevated levels of *Cladosporium* and *Aspergillus*. Conversely, arid regions, such as the southwestern states, have a higher prevalence of *Alternaria*. Indoor fungal allergens, while less influenced by seasonality, tend to increase in poorly ventilated or water-damaged homes.

Emerging Challenges and Climate Influence

Climate change is altering the dynamics of fungal aeroallergens. Warmer temperatures and increased humidity create favorable conditions for mold growth and spore production, potentially extending the duration of fungal allergy seasons. Extreme weather events, such as hurricanes and floods, exacerbate indoor mold problems by causing water damage to buildings, leading to higher exposure levels.

Health Implications and Monitoring

Fungal aeroallergens are a critical public health concern due to their association with severe respiratory diseases and asthma exacerbations. Monitoring and identifying fungal spores in the environment are essential for understanding exposure risks and implementing mitigation strategies. Advances in aerobiology, such as molecular techniques for fungal identification, are enhancing the ability to detect and quantify fungal allergens in the air, contributing to improved disease management and prevention efforts.

By understanding the diversity, distribution, and dynamics of fungal aeroallergens, researchers and healthcare professionals can better address the growing challenges posed by these ubiquitous allergens in the United States.

Meteorological Variables

Meteorological factors significantly influence the release, dispersion, and persistence of aeroallergens in the atmosphere. These variables, including temperature, humidity, wind speed, precipitation, and solar radiation, interact dynamically with biological and environmental processes to shape aeroallergen concentrations and distribution patterns. Understanding these relationships is critical for predicting allergen exposure risks and developing strategies to manage allergic diseases.

Temperature

Temperature is one of the most important meteorological factors affecting aeroallergens. It directly impacts the growth and reproductive cycles of allergen-producing organisms such as plants and fungi. Warmer temperatures often accelerate the development of plants and lead to earlier and prolonged pollen seasons. For example, tree pollination in temperate regions has advanced significantly in recent decades due to global warming, increasing exposure risks. Similarly, fungal growth and spore release are temperature-sensitive, with many fungal species showing optimal sporulation within specific temperature ranges.

Humidity

Humidity influences aeroallergens by affecting their production, release, and viability. High humidity levels promote the growth of mold and dust mites, increasing indoor allergen concentrations. However, excessive moisture can reduce the release of airborne pollen and fungal spores by causing them to clump or adhere to surfaces. Conversely, low humidity levels, often associated with dry and windy conditions, can enhance the dispersion of lightweight allergenic particles such as pollen, allowing them to travel long distances.

Wind Speed and Direction

Wind plays a critical role in dispersing aeroallergens across geographic regions. Strong winds can carry pollen grains and fungal spores far from their sources, increasing the exposure of populations in distant areas. The direction and variability of wind patterns also influence allergen distribution, as they determine the trajectory of airborne particles. For instance, coastal regions often experience allergen transport from inland areas, while urban environments may have reduced allergen levels due to wind shielding by buildings.

Precipitation

Rainfall has a dual effect on aeroallergen dynamics. Light to moderate rain can remove allergens from the air by washing them onto surfaces, temporarily reducing atmospheric concentrations. However, heavy rainfall, particularly during thunderstorms, can enhance aeroallergen exposure. Thunderstorm-associated winds and turbulence can rupture pollen grains, releasing allergenic subparticles that are small enough to penetrate deep into the respiratory tract, triggering severe allergic reactions such as thunderstorm asthma.

Solar Radiation

Solar radiation affects aeroallergens by influencing plant photosynthesis and the timing of pollen release. Many plants rely on diurnal cycles of light and temperature to regulate their reproductive processes, with peak pollen release often occurring in the morning when sunlight intensity increases. Additionally, ultraviolet (UV) radiation can degrade allergenic proteins, reducing their potency in some cases. However, in urban environments, high levels of air pollution can interact with UV radiation to modify allergen structures, potentially increasing their allergenicity.

Interactions Between Variables

Meteorological variables rarely act in isolation; their combined effects often determine aeroallergen behavior. For example, high temperatures and low humidity levels during the summer can lead to peak pollen and spore concentrations, while the onset of a rainstorm may abruptly reduce these levels. Seasonal variations in climate also influence the relative importance of different meteorological factors, with temperature dominating during spring and summer, and humidity and precipitation playing larger roles in autumn and winter.

The interplay between meteorological variables and aeroallergens underscores the need for integrated monitoring systems and predictive models. Enhanced aeroallergen surveillance is essential for identifying existing patterns and detecting shifts over time. By combining allergen data with weather forecasts, it is possible to develop accurate exposure risk assessments, inform public health strategies, and support individuals in managing allergic conditions.

Impact of Climate Change on Aeroallergens

Climate change is profoundly altering the dynamics of aeroallergens, with significant implications for allergic diseases and public health. Rising global temperatures, changes in precipitation patterns, and increasing levels of atmospheric carbon dioxide (CO_2) are driving shifts in the production, distribution, and potency of aeroallergens. These changes are expected to exacerbate allergen exposure and the burden of respiratory and allergic conditions worldwide.

Increased Pollen Production

Elevated atmospheric CO_2 levels, a primary driver of climate change, stimulate photosynthesis and enhance the growth of plants. This increased biomass often translates into higher pollen production. Studies have shown that plants such as ragweed (*Ambrosia artemisiifolia*), a major source of allergenic pollen, produce significantly more pollen under elevated CO_2 conditions. Furthermore, climate change is extending the growing seasons of many plants, leading to longer periods of pollen release and prolonged exposure for individuals with pollen allergies.

Earlier and Longer Pollen Seasons

Rising temperatures are causing plants to flower and release pollen earlier in the year. This phenomenon, often referred to as the "advancement of phenology," has been documented in numerous regions, particularly in temperate climates. For example, tree pollen seasons in parts of Europe and North America are starting earlier and lasting longer, increasing cumulative allergen exposure. Prolonged pollen seasons not only heighten the risk of sensitization in vulnerable populations but also exacerbate symptoms in individuals with pre-existing allergies.

Changes in Allergen Potency

Climate change also affects the allergenic potential of aeroallergens. Elevated CO_2 and ozone levels can alter the protein composition of pollen grains, increasing their allergenicity. For instance, ragweed plants grown under higher CO_2 conditions produce pollen with higher concentrations of allergenic proteins, such as Amb a 1. These changes can intensify the severity of allergic reactions and complicate the management of allergic diseases. Over the last 20 to 30 years there has been an estimated 21% increase in pollen concentrations across North America that is highly correlated with warming. Additionally, interactions between pollen and air pollutants, which are exacerbated by climate change, can further modify allergenic proteins, making them more potent triggers of immune responses.

Shifts in Geographic Distribution

Climate change is reshaping the geographic distribution of allergenic plants and fungi. Rising temperatures and altered precipitation patterns enable the northward migration of species such as ragweed into regions that were previously unsuitable for their growth. This expansion introduces new populations to allergen exposure, potentially increasing the prevalence of allergies in these areas. Similarly, warmer and wetter conditions promote the growth of mold and fungi, raising the levels of airborne fungal spores in regions with high humidity.

Thunderstorm-Related Aeroallergen Events

Climate change is associated with an increase in the frequency and intensity of extreme weather events, including thunderstorms. These storms can exacerbate aeroallergen exposure by dispersing pollen grains, rupturing them into smaller allergenic fragments, and generating strong wind currents that transport allergens over large distances. Thunderstorm asthma, a severe allergic reaction triggered by such events, has become more frequent in regions experiencing climatic instability, posing significant public health challenges.

Cumulative Health Impacts

The cumulative effects of climate change on aeroallergens are likely to result in a greater burden of allergic diseases, including asthma, allergic rhinitis, and atopic dermatitis. Populations in urban areas may be particularly vulnerable due to the combined effects of climate change, pollution, and limited access to green spaces that could mitigate allergen exposure. Furthermore, the increased allergen burden may disproportionately affect low-income communities with limited healthcare access and greater exposure to environmental stressors.

Addressing the impact of climate change on aeroallergens requires integrated strategies, including enhanced monitoring of allergen levels, predictive modeling of future trends, and public health initiatives. A comprehensive approach will allow researchers and policymakers to develop targeted interventions to reduce the health burden associated with allergic diseases in a rapidly changing climate.

Conclusions

Aeroallergens play a central role in the development and exacerbation of allergic diseases, significantly impacting public health and quality of life worldwide. These airborne particles, derived from diverse biological sources such as pollen, fungal spores, dust mites, and animal dander, are influenced by complex interactions between environmental, biological, and meteorological factors. Understanding these interactions is essential for advancing the field of allergology and mitigating the burden of allergen-related diseases.

The diversity of aeroallergens highlights the importance of regional and seasonal considerations in assessing allergen exposure. In the United States, the contribution of tree, grass, and weed pollen varies across different geographic regions, influenced by climate and vegetation patterns. Similarly, fungal spores and indoor allergens exhibit unique environmental and seasonal dynamics, emphasizing the need for localized strategies in monitoring and management. As climate change alters these patterns, it becomes increasingly critical to study and predict changes in aeroallergen prevalence, potency, and distribution to anticipate future public health challenges.

Advances in aerobiology have significantly enhanced our ability to detect, quantify, and understand aeroallergens. Modern sampling techniques, coupled with molecular and immunological analyses, provide detailed insights into allergen composition and exposure dynamics. These tools are invaluable for identifying emerging allergens, assessing health risks, and developing precise interventions. Integrated monitoring systems, incorporating meteorological data and predictive modeling, hold great promise for improving allergen forecasts and empowering individuals to manage their exposure effectively.

The growing recognition of the impact of climate change on aeroallergens underscores the need for multidisciplinary approaches to address this evolving issue. Rising temperatures, increased atmospheric carbon dioxide levels, and extreme weather events are reshaping the dynamics of aeroallergen release and dispersion. Collaborative efforts between researchers, public health officials, and policymakers are crucial to develop adaptive strategies that mitigate the health effects of these changes, especially in vulnerable populations.

In conclusion, the study of aeroallergens is an interdisciplinary endeavor at the intersection of biology, environmental science, and public health. By fostering a deeper understanding of aeroallergen sources, dynamics, and impacts, we can develop effective tools and strategies to reduce allergen exposure and improve health outcomes. Continued research, innovation, and public health initiatives will be vital for addressing the challenges posed by aeroallergens in the context of a rapidly changing environment.

Chapter 3
Allergic Rhinitis

Amna Hassan and Jonathan A. Bernstein

Introduction

Allergic rhinitis (AR) isdefined by intermittent or persistent symptoms of sneezing, itchy eyes, ears, nose, rhinorrhea and nasal congestion with positive specific IgE testing to aeroallergens that correlates with the occurrence of symptoms, It is estimated to affect approximately 15% of people in the United States andapproximately 500million worldwide.(The prevalence of AR may be as high as 30% if diagnosis is based nasal symptoms alone. Allergic rhinitis is associated with the presence of co-morbid conditions including asthma, eczema, chronic or recurrent sinusitis, cough, headache and sleep disturbances. Therefore, it is not surprising that AR significantly impacts the patient's quality of life and is associated with significant direct or indirect healthcare costs. To minimize the burden of AR on patients, it is important to diagnose and treat this condition properly.

A. Hassan
Department of Internal Medicine, Division of Rheumatology, University of Cincinnati College of Medicine, Allergy and Immunology, Cincinnati, OH, USA

J. A. Bernstein (✉)
Department of Internal Medicine, Division of Rheumatology, Allergy and Immunology, Partner Advanced Allergy Services, LLC, Partner Bernstein Clinical Research Center, University of Cincinnati College of Medicine, Cincinnati, OH, USA
e-mail: Bernstja@ucmail.uc.edu

M. Mahmoudi (ed.), *Treatment and Management of Allergic Rhinitis*,
https://doi.org/10.1007/978-3-031-88107-7_3

Burden of Disease

National telephone and on-line survey studies interviewing adults with AR reported a significant association of their AR symptoms on quality of life (QoL), sleep, work and school productivity, comorbid conditions, in addition to poor efficacy and tolerability of pharmacologic treatment.A2012 survey of 2500 adults from North America, Latin America, and the Asia-Pacific region with AR, reported up to 50% reported symptoms associated with at least a moderate effect on their daily life and up to 25% reported sleep disturbances. A 2017 US questionnaire surveyenrolled 500 adults and 501 childrenrandomly selected from aHarris poll data meeting inclusion criteria for seasonal allergic rhinoconjunctivitis. Over50% of respondents experienceddaily seasonal symptoms and 75–80% reportedmoderate to severe symptoms that significantly affected their quality of life. Allergic rhinitis was also found to be significantly associated with fatigue in adults and children due to poor sleep quality caused by uncontrolled symptomsand medicationside effects, impaired physical and social functioning, cognitive and memory impairment leading to anxiety, depression, and work or school absenteeism or presenteeism. A recent cost analysis of AR revealed an annualmean total cost per patient for rhinitis management including testing, diagnostic procedures, clinic visits and surgery was $281. Based on the prevalence of chronic rhinitis the total estimated cost was $3.3 billion not including medications which were estimated to cost $1.3 billion a year.

Pathogenesis

Allergic rhinitis patients have impairment of their nasal epithelial barrier which makes them more susceptible to aeroallergen sensitizationto protease-containing allergens (e.g. dust mites, mold spores), or from non-specific inflammatory responses frominfectious agents (e.g. bacteria, virus), and air pollutants (e.g. particulate matter, diesel exhaust particles, tobacco smoke) (Fig. 3.1) When an allergen entersthe nose and attaches to the mucus membrane, it is processed by antigen presenting cells (e.g., dendritic cells), resulting in activation of naïve T cellsthat differentiate to Th2 cells capable of releasing Type 2 cytokines (e.g. IL-4, IL-5, IL-13) that leads toB cellproduction of specific immunoglobulin E to the allergen(sIgE). The sIgE antibody binds to high affinity IgE receptors (FcεRII) on mast cells, skin Langerhans cells, monocytes, and basophils. Upon reexposure, the sensitizing allergen is recognized by the sIgE antigen binding region of the IgE molecule on the IgE receptor,resulting in mast cell activation and release of bioactive mediators including histamine, leukotrienes, and platelet activating factor that cause physiologic changes resulting in the classic symptoms of AR which includes sneezing, itching, rhinorrhea and nasal congestion. In addition, epithelial disruption leads to innate lymphoid responses and activation of neurogenic pathways that further enhance the inflammatory response in AR.

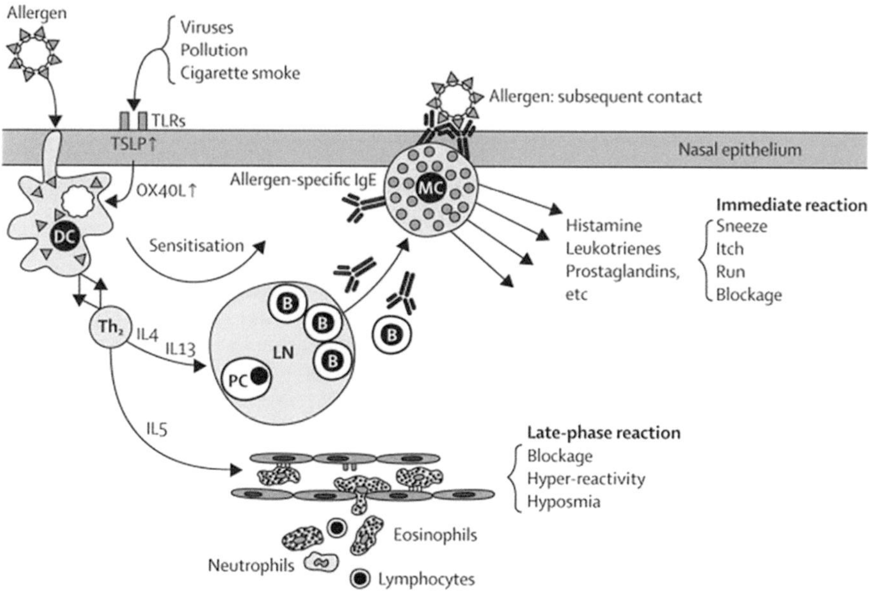

Fig. 3.1 The pathogenesis of allergic rhinitis. (Source: Greiner et al. 2011)

Differential Diagnosis

The differential diagnosis of AR includes localized AR, non-allergic rhinitis (NAR), mixed rhinitis which is rhinitis characterized by allergic and non-allergic triggers, occupational rhinitis, infectious rhinitis, and medication induced rhinitis (Table 3.1). Localized AR clinically presents like AR, but diagnosis is confirmed by nasal provocation to the suspected specific allergen as specific IgE testing to aeroallergens are-negative. Non-allergic rhinitis, the most common form being vasomotor rhinitis (VMR), presents primarily with nasal congestion, post-nasal drainage, ear plugging secondary to eustachian tube dysfunction, headache, sinus pressure and pain triggered by chemicals, irritants and weather changes and patients have negative specific IgE testing to aeroallergens.Occupational rhinitis is caused by workplace exposures that can either elicit allergic or irritant induced nasal symptoms and is often a precursor to the development of occupational asthma. The most common causes of OR are chemical cleaning agents or sterilizing agents that are widely used in the custodian or healthcare industries. Infectious rhinitis is caused primarily by viral upper respiratory infections.Medication induced rhinitis occurs secondary to different types of medications including non-steroidal anti-inflammatory agents, anti-hypertensives such as beta-blockers and calcium channel blockers and estrogen containing hormonesandis believed to cause vasodilation through neurogenic pathways.

Table 3.1 Differential diagnosis and characteristics of allergic rhinitis

Differential diagnosis of allergic rhinitis	Definition	Clinical clues	Mechanism	Treatment
Seasonal allergic rhinitis	Sensitization to seasonal pollen allergens	Childhood onset Seasonal symptoms of itching, sneezing, rhinorrhea and nasal congestion Family history	IgE-mediated	SGAH, INCS, INAH, LTRA IT
Perennial allergic rhinitis	Sensitization to year roundallergens like animals and dust mites	Symptoms around cats, dogs, dust mite that improves with avoidance Symptoms of itching, sneezing, rhinorrhea but persistent nasal congestion, and post-nasal drainage	IgE-mediated	SGAH, INCS, INAH, LTRA, AIT
Localized (entopic) allergic rhinitis	Symptoms of perennial or seasonal rhinitis, with negative skin or serum sIgE testing; confirmed byspecific nasal allergen provocation test (NAPT)	Symptoms like classical allergic presentation, but skin testing negative Consider NAPT if high suspicion for this condition	IgE-mediated	SGAH, INCS, INAH, LTRA, AIT
Vasomotor rhinitis	The most common form of non-allergic rhinitis also referred to as non-allergic rhinopathy	Year roundnasal congestion and post-nasal drainage; no seasonality Associated frequently with eustachian tube dysfunction Onset later in life No family history Triggered by fragrances and other irritants	Neuropathic)	INAH, INCS, anti-cholinergic agents to control drainage
Non-allergic rhinitis with eosinophil syndrome (NARES)	Year round non-allergic rhinitis with increased nasal eosinophils	Responsive to INCS and no evidence of nasal polyps	Neuropathic	INAH, INCS, anti-cholinergic to control drainage

(continued)

Table 3.1 (continued)

Differential diagnosis of allergic rhinitis	Definition	Clinical clues	Mechanism	Treatment
Occupational rhinitis (aka work-related rhinitis)	Rhinitis induced by occupational environmental exposures; need to differentiate from work exacerbated rhinitis which is pre-existing rhinitisworsenedby workplace exposures)	No prior history of rhinitis Symptoms worse atworkand improveaway from work.	High molecular weight agents—IgE-mediated Low molecular weight agents—IgE or non-IgE (neuropathic)	Treatment similar to either AR or NAR depending on whether inciting agent is sensitizing or irritant.
Drug-induced rhinitis	Pharmacologic effect—	Common medications associated with congestion include topical nasal decongestants, oral contraceptives, nonsteroidal anti-inflammatory drugs, antihypertensive medications (β-blockers)	May be neurogenic or related to MGPRX2 mediated	Avoidance
Infectious rhinitis	Can be acute or chronic. Mostly viral but can lead to a bacterial infection Fungal infections should be considered especially in immunocompromised patients	Suspect bacterial when symptoms persist >10 days	Innate immune response mediated	Viral- self-limiting Bacterial-antibiotics Fungal-surgical debridement

SGAH second generation antihistamines, *LTRA* leukotriene receptor antagonist, *INCS* intranasal corticosteroids, *INAH* intranasal antihistamines, *AIT* llergen immunotherapy

Risk Factors

Risk factors for AR include changes in the normal gut microbiome at birth. Factors that maintain a normal gut microbiome and are believed to protect against developing Type 2 allergic inflammation includenormal vaginal delivery, normal gestational age, breastfeeding, early exposure to pets in the home (e.g. dogs), two or more siblings in the home and a rural environment. Other factors that increase risk for allergy include family history, eczema as a baby, early antibiotic exposure and urban living associated with decreased biodiversity,

Comorbid Conditions

Allergic rhinitis patients are at increased risk for a spectrum of co-morbid conditions includingallergic conjunctivitis, acute and chronic sinusitis, otitis media in children, eustachian tube dysfunction, chronic cough due to post-nasal drainage and asthma. Many of these complications are the result of inflammation that block passages of the lacrimal duct and sinus ostia that empty into the nose leading to symptoms. There are several explanations for the association between AR and asthmabut it is believed to be primarily secondary to a bidirectional inflammatory interaction between the upper and lower respiratory tracts and neuroreflex mechanisms.

Patients with AR may also present with chronic rhinosinusitis with or without nasal polyposis (~30%), migraine or tension type headaches (~13.5%) and sleep disturbances such as obstructive sleep apnea (~25%) which may improve after treating AR.

Diagnosis

PreviouslyPatients with SAR typically report anterior rhinorrhea (runny nose), nasal itching, repeated sneezing, and watery, itchy eyes whereas PAR patients experience more nasal congestion and post-nasal drainage., Arhinitis questionnaire study that analyzed chronic rhinitis patientsfound that the absence of seasonal (e.g. spring) outdoor symptoms), parental history of allergy, symptoms around cats, occurrence of symptoms around perfumes and fragrances and age greater than 35 atsymptom onset were predictive for NAR. These questions are important for ascertaining whether patients with AR have NAR or an NAR component as up to 50% of patients with chronic rhinitis have MR.

Diagnostic testing for AR performed by an allergy specialist includes either skin prick tests (SPT) or sIgE serologic testingto relevant aeroallergens in their geographic location. Skin prick testing involves placing a drop of a specific allergen on the patient's back or forearm and pricking it with a bifurcated needle which will elicit a wheal and flare reaction within 15 min if the patient is sensitized. Specific IgE serologic testing to specific aeroallergens utilizes an enzymatic assay (i.e., Immunocap™) to assess for sensitization.Skin prict testing has an 85% sensitivity and 77% specificity for confirming AR and studies have demonstrated good correlation between skin prick testing and Immunocap sIgE. There are nuances for performing and interpreting these tests that should be understood to avoid misinterpretation of results. For example, all patients undergoing SPTs should be tested for dermographism which can elicit false positive results and be told to avoid medications that block H1-receptors for several days before testing which can cause false negative results. Regardless of which approach is used, the testing panels include representative trees, grassand weed pollens, outdoor (Alternaria) and indoor (e.g., Aspergillus niger, Penicillium notatum) molds, dust mite, cat, dog, and cockroach. Any positive test should correlate with the patient's symptoms when exposed to the allergen. A positive skin test alone is not diagnostic of AR. If SPTs are negative, placing a select number ofintracutaneous tests where a small volume of the suspected allergen is injected underneath the forearm skin toelicit a wheal and flare response within 10–15 min, can be performed if there is strong suspicion for sensitization to an allergen that was negative by SPT. However, these tests are more sensitive resulting in false positive results and should therefore be interpreted with caution. There are many unproven, non-validated allergen diagnostic testing that is being performed such as skin end-point titration (Rinkel Method), provocation-neutralization, antigen leukocyte cellular antibody test (ALCAT), and electrodermal testing that are not recommended for the diagnosis of AR.

As mentioned previously, approximately 30% of AR patients may also have asthma which may not be readily recognized by patients as they don't always experience typical asthma symptoms. Therefore, all AR patientsshould be questioned for symptoms related to asthma and assessed objectively with spirometry to measure the forced expiratory volume in the first second of exhalation (FEV1) to determine if there is airway obstruction and /or reversibility after short-acting beta-2-agonists. A 12% or greaterincrease in FEV1 or an absolute increase of 200 ml or greaterin FEV1 is supportive of an asthma diagnosis. If there is no evidence of reversibility but high suspicion for asthma then a bronchoprovocation test such as a methacholine challenge should be obtained to rule in or out airway hyperresponsiveness representative of smooth muscle dysfunction, a central feature of asthma. It is important to establish an objective diagnosis of asthma especially if patients are undergoing allergen immunotherapy for their AR as underlying undiagnosed, uncontrolled asthma is a risk factor for fatal or near fatal injection reactions. Peripheral blood eosinophils, which correlate with eosinophils in the lung, is also a helpful adjunctive test for assessing for asthma.

Treatment

Environmental Interventions

Avoidance of allergens to which the patient is sensitized should be implemented in the home and workplace. There have been many studies investigating the effectiveness of indoor allergen remediation and some interventions are more strongly recommended than others. Pollen allergic patients should keep windows closed and run the air conditioning during the warmer times of the year to reduce indoor exposure to outdoor aeroallergens. For dust mites which have been found in reservoirs such as pillows, mattresses, box springs, carpeting and upholstered furniture, placing dust mite impermeable encasements on bedding,carpet vacuuming at least 1–2 times a week orreplacement of carpets from main activity rooms with hardwood or tileflooring has been found to significantly reduce symptoms in dust mite sensitized

AR patients. Maintaining indoor humidity between 30% and 50% using air-conditioning or an external dehumidifier also decreases dust mite growth. For sensitized pet owners who are unwilling to remove these animals for the home, keeping pets out of the bedroom and using high efficiency particulate air (HEPA) filters in the bedroom and main activity rooms has been found to be helpful in reducing airborne pet allergen levels. Extermination in conjunction with thorough cleaning has been found to be helpful in eliminating cockroach and rodent allergen levels.In general, the most effective environmental control practice involves utilizing amulti-componentintervention andmaintenance approach which can be associated with poor adherence and significant costs. Finally, it is important to reduce or eliminate indoor sources of air pollutants that can worsen AR. These pollutants include nitrogen dioxide (e.g. source: gas stoves, kerosene heaters), ozone (e.g. source: electrical appliances), and chemical volatile organic compounds (e.g. source: cleaning agents, paints, solvents). It is essential that home and work air -filtration systems are well maintained to ensuresufficient indoor and outdoor air exchange necessary to maintain good indoor air quality and that furnace filters are regularly changed.

Pharmacotherapy

An algorithmic treatment approach has been recommended in recent rhinitis guidelines. Treatment selection is based on severity of disease and it is recommended that treatment is increased or decreased based on symptom control (Tables 3.2 and 3.3). For SAR, therapy may be discontinuedafter the season is over, however, patients with PARoften require therapy year-round to control symptoms and prevent co-morbid complications.

Guidelines recommend as first-line treatment for intermittent AR oral H1-second-generation antihistamines (SGAH), such as fexofenadine, cetirizine, levocetirizine and desloratadine which are all over-the-counter (OTC) except for desloratadine. In addition, intranasal antihistamines (INAH) such as azelastine and olopatadine (OLO), or intranasal corticosteroids(INCS) such as fluticasone, triamcinolone, budesonide and mometasone,which are all OTC, except for olopatadine,are also recommended for intermittent AR like SAR. All these medications can be used during the season and then discontinued when the season is over. For moderate to severe AR, INCS consideredthe first line topical therapies.Patients need to be properly instructed on how to use agents, angling the spray away from the nasal septum to prevent septal erosions, ulcerations and nasal bleeding. Some INCSs have also been demonstrated to control allergic conjunctivitis associated with AR.There have been reports of INCS increasing ocular pressure in patients with glaucoma which in some patients may preclude their use. Intranasal antihistamines are approved for AR and NAR and are well tolerated with few side effects but in some patients may cause excessive dryness with nose bleeding, sedation and less commonly. Second generation antihistamines can be used adjunctively to INCS with or without INAH safely

Table 3.2 Algorithm for treatment of intermittentand persistent AR for patients ages 12 years and older

Intermittent allergic rhinitis treatment 12 years and older	
Mild symptoms	**Moderate to severe symptoms**
First line: Oral SGAH or INAH; second line: Oral SGAH+PSE[a] or INCS; can an intranasal decongestant to INCS for moderate to severe nasal congestion[b]	First line: Oral SGAH or INAH; second line: INCS; third line: Combination INCS+INAH; can add oral PSE[a] or intranasal decongestant[b] for moderate to severe nasal congestion
	SGAH+INCS and LTRA not recommended for first line treatment[a]
Persistent allergic rhinitis treatment 12 years and older	
Mild symptoms	**Moderate to severe symptoms**
First line; INCS; second line: Add SGAH or INAH; third line: Can use SGAH/PSE or intranasal decongestion in conjunction with INCS up to 4–6 weeks as tolerated for severe congestion; fourth line: Can add intranasal cromolyn sodium	First line: INCS + INAH back-to-back or INCS/INAH combination
LTRA not recommended for first line treatment[a]	SGAH/INCS and SGAH/PSE are not recommended as first line treatments[a]

Adapted from Rhinitis 2020 Guidelines
LTRA leukotriene receptor antagonist, *SGAH* second generation antihistamine, *INAH* intranasal antihistamine, *INCS* intranasal corticosteroid
[a]PSE—pseudoephedrine should be used with caution due to known side effects of increased blood pressure, palpitations, insomnia, and restlessness
[b]Intranasal decongestants can be used safely in conjunction with INCS for up to 4–6 weeks without rebound congestion

as they are generally well tolerated and don't bind to cholinergic receptors or cross the blood-brain-barrier, which makes them lessdrying and sedating. However, for AR, some studies have suggested that improvement of symptoms with an INCS is as effective as monotherapy as combination therapy with an INCS and SGAHIf patients don't respond to these medications, then they may have a more complex form of AR associated with NAR (MR)or have structural abnormalities that impede their effectiveness. In these circumstances, it may be necessary to further assess with a sinus CT scan or nasal endoscopy. Treatment of children ≥ 6 years of age does not differ from adults except for medication dosing.

It is not recommended that clinicians use repeated injections with intramuscular-glucocorticoidsto treatSAR or PAR, due to theirwell-documented cumulative side effects over time (Lugogo et al. 2022). An exception would be use of a brief course of short course of high dose oral glucocorticoids (35–40 mg for 5–7 days) for an SAR exacerbation that isn't well controlled with conventional topical or systemic agents. Even though most AR medications are available over the counter, use of these medications by patients should be supervised by their physician to ensure they are being used properly to optimize efficacy and minimize side effects. Adjunctive use of isotonic or hypertonic saline irrigation solutionsand nutraceuticalssuch asintranasal capsaicin have been shown to have some benefit in the treatment of AR.

Table 3.3 Medications for allergic rhinitis

Therapy	Examples of adult dosing	Onset of action	Maximal effect	Efficacy	Adverse effects
Intranasal corticosteroid/ intranasal antihistamine combination	Fluticasone (50ug)/Azelastine (137ug)/per actuation 1 puff each nostril twice daily, Mometasone (25ug)/Olopatadine (665ug) 2 puffs each nostril twice daily	5 min	2 weeks or longer	More effective than INCS or INAH monotherapy and placebo in terms of improved nasal symptoms, ocular symptoms, and quality of life (Chitsuthipakorn et al. 2022; Lugogo et al. 2022)	Nasal irritation, epistaxis Increased cost for combination formulation
INCS- alcohol based	Fluticasone propionate (50ug) 1–2 puffs each nostril daily	2–12 h	2 weeks	First line for moderate/severe seasonal allergic rhinitis, and for persistent, allergic/nonallergic rhinitis >15 years old. (strong recommendation, high certainty of evidence) (Meltzer et al. 2012)	Nasal irritation and epistaxis (risk increased with alcohol-based formulations)
Intranasal corticosteroids- aqueous based	Fluticasone furoate (27.5ug) 1–2 puffs each nostril once daily	8 h	2–4 weeks	Recent metanalysis showed superiority to placebo but similar efficacy amongst INCS for improving total nasal and ocular symptom scores (Soe et al. 2023) Non-alcohol based nasal corticosteroids are associated with less nasal irritation than alcohol based formualtions.	Short term use may decrease short term growth velocity, but no long effect on long term growth velocity. Use lowest effective dose and monitor growth Theoretical concern for increased intraocular pressure- use with caution in patients with glaucoma, cataracts
	Mometasone furoate (50ug) 2 puffs each nostril once daily	2–5 h	4 weeks		
	Ciclesonide (50ug) 2 puffs each nostril once daily	1–6 h	2–4 weeks		
	Budesonide (32ug) 1–4 puffs each nostril once daily	3–8 h	2–4 weeks		
	Triamcinolone acetonide (55ug) 1–2 puffs each nostril once daily	12 h	2–4 weeks		
Intranasal antihistamines	Azelastine .1% (137ug) 1–2 puffs each nostril twice daily for PAR and VMR Azelastine .15% (205.5ug) 2 puffs each nostil daily for SAR and twice daily for PAR	15 mins	1 day to 4 weeks for both	First line for seasonal allergic, intermittent, and non-allergic rhinitis (strong recommendation, high certainty of evidence) (Meltzer et al. 2012)	Bitter taste (greater in azelastine) Nasal irritation, epistaxis
	Olopatadine .6% (665ug) 2 puffs each nostril twice a day for SAR	30 min			

Intranasal anticholinergic	Ipratropium bromide .03% (21ug) 2 puffs each nostril 2–3 times a day for PAR and NAR Ipratropium bromide .06% (42ug) 2 puff each nostril 4 times a day for SAR and 3–4 times a day for the common cold	15 min	1 h	Consider for treating anterior rhinorrhea in non-allergic rhinitis (moderate evidence), and perennial rhinitis (low level) (Meltzer et al. 2012)	Nasal irritation, epistaxis Caution with glaucoma
Second generation Oral antihistamines	Desloratadine 5 mg once daily	30–90 min	1–8 days	More effective than placebo in alleviating allergic rhinitis symptoms; less effective than INCS (Meltzer et al. 2012)	Minimal side effect profile; may cause nasal/ocular dryness For renal failure, can use loratadine and first-generation antihistamine, diphenhydramine For hepatic failure, can use first generation antihistamine, diphenhydramine, or cetirizine although dose may have to be reduced
	Levocetirizine 2.5 mg to 5 mg once daily	45 min			
	Cetirizine 5-10 mg once daily as needed	60 min			
	Loratadine 10 mg once daily as needed	60–75 min			
	Fexofenadine 180 mg once daily as needed	60 min			
Oral first-generation antihistamines	Diphenhydramine 25-50 mg every 4–6 h as needed	20–30 min	1 h	No existing DBPC trials to evaluate therapeutic efficacy of first vs second generation oral antihistamines	Attributed to non-specific cholinergic and alpha-adrenergic receptor binding. Can lead to sedation, increased risk of dementia, dry eyes, dry mouth, urinary retention, dose dependent tachycardia and risk of arrhythmias
Intranasal decongestant	Oxymetazoline .05% 2–3 puffs every 10–12 h as needed; if used longer than 5–7 days should be administered with an INCS	<10 min	Within 60 mins	For short term benefit of nasal congestion	Rhinitis medicamentosa as soon as 3 days after use. Studies show coadministration of INCS helps to prevent rhinitis medicamentosa for 4 weeks

(continued)

Table 3.3 (continued)

Therapy	Examples of adult dosing	Onset of action	Maximal effect	Efficacy	Adverse effects
Oral SGAH with decongestant	Loratadine 5 mg/pseudoephedrine 120 mg every 12 h as needed Loratadine 10 mg/pseudoephedrine 240ug once daily as needed Fexofenadine 60 mg/pseudoephedrine 120 mg every 12 h as needed Fexofenadine 180 mg/pseudoephedrine 240ug once daily as needed Cetirizine 5 mg/pseudoephedrine 120 mg every 12 h as needed Cetirizine 10 mg/pseudoephedrine 240ug once daily as needed	30 min	Unknown	More effective than individual components	
LTRA	Montelukast 10 mg once a day	Within 5 h	By week two	Montelukast more effective than placebo for improving daytime nasal score, nighttime nasal symptoms, and composite symptom scores (Krishnamoorthy et al. 2020). Oral antihistamine are superior to montelukast in improving daytime nasal symptoms and composite symptom scores, daytime eye symptoms and quality of life. Montelukast is superior to oral antihistamine in improving nighttime nasal symptoms (Krishnamoorthy et al. 2020)	Black box warning neuropsychiatric side effects
Intranasal mast cell stabilizer	Cromolyn sodium (5.2 mg) one puff each nostril 3–4 times a day	2 weeks	At least 2 weeks	Improves symptoms of SAR vs placebo, but not with PAR; may be most helpful immediately before allergen exposure (very low level of evidence) (Meltzer et al. 2012)	Low side effect profile; safe in pregnancy

CS corticosteroid, *AH* antihistamine, *LTRA* leukotriene receptor antagonist, *INCS* intranasal corticosteroid, *INAH* intranasal antihistamine, *SAR* seasonal allergic rhinitis, *PAR* perennial allergic rhinitis, *VMR* vasomotor rhinitis, *NAR* non-allergic rhinitis

Immunotherapy

Patients with persistent AR symptoms despite optimal pharmacologic therapy and avoidance measures can be considered for allergen immunotherapy (AIT),which has been shown to induce tolerance and prevent co-morbid conditions such as sinusitis and asthma in children and adults. Similar to pharmacotherapy, proper patient selection s with allergen sensitization that correlates with symptoms upon exposure to the sensitizing allergens who do not want to depend on medications or don't tolerate medications for symptom control and are willing to adhere to AIT is essential for optimal outcomes.

Subcutaneousimmunotherapy (SCIT) and sublingual immunotherapy (SLIT) are both FDA approved forms of AIT. Subcutaneous IT works by increasing regulatory T cells which increase cytokines like IL-10 that promote tolerance and the production of allergen-specific IgG blocking antibodies, however, other mechanisms yet to be fully characterized may also be involved. Subligualimmunotherapy is believed to work through similar mechanisms but may also involve oral dendritic cells that also promote tolerance. Subcutaneous immunotherapyshould be administered by an experienced Allergist or Otolaryngology specialist in an office setting where emergency medications (e.g., epinephrine) is readily available should a systemic anaphylactic reaction occur. It is possible to administer SCIT using conventional protocols with slow build to a maintenance dose that takes up to 6 months. Alternative rush or cluster protocols allow faster build up to higher concentrations over 3–4 visits and have been demonstrated to be safe if patients are pretreated with SGAH, leukotriene antagonists and oral glucocorticoids to prevent systemic reactions. If effective, AIT is recommended to continue up to 3–5 years but may require a longer course of therapy for some patients. It is recommended to take periodic breaks in therapy over 2–3 months during the patient's worst season to determine if AIT needs to be continued or can be discontinued. The estimated 5-year cost of AIT is approximately $5000. In contrast to SCIT, SLIT can be safely self-administered at home after the first dose is administered in a medical office under the supervision of a medical professional. The risk of a systemic reaction to SCIT is approximately 1 per 1000 injections (0.1%) and life-threatening anaphylaxis occur in 1/160,000 injections. Patients at risk for systemic reactions should have an IM or intranasal epinephrine self-injector. Approximately 50% of patients treated with SLIT mayexperienceoral palatal itching which can be uncomfortable but has not been associated with progression to laryngeal edema or a systemic reaction. It is the responsibility of the physician prescribing SCIT or SLIT to educate the patients about the efficacy and safety of these treatment modalities.

Conclusions

Allergic rhinitis is a prevalent chronic disease that has a significant health and economic burden on society. If diagnosed and treated properly, AR has an excellent prognosis and other comorbid illnesses such as sinus infections and asthma can be prevented or improved. The clinician needs to differentiate AR from other forms of chronic rhinitis which may have overlapping causes and treatments but have distinct nuances that are necessary to recognize to ensure optimal outcomes. Treatment of AR includes a combination of avoidance of triggers, medications and if indicated allergen immunotherapy. Early diagnosis of patients with AR based on risk factors will help to significantly reduce its associated disease morbidity and health care costs.

Suggested Reading

Alromaih S, Alsagaf L, Aloraini N, Alrasheed A, Alroqi A, Aloulah M, et al. Drug-induced rhinitis: narrative review. Ear Nose Throat J. 2022;1455613221141214

Alvaro-Lozano M, Akdis CA, Akdis M, Alviani C, Angier E, Arasi S, et al. EAACI allergen immunotherapy user's guide. Pediatr Allergy Immunol. 2020;31(Suppl 25):1–101.

Arlian LG, Platts-Mills TA. The biology of dust mites and the remediation of mite allergens in allergic disease. J Allergy Clin Immunol. 2001;107(3 Suppl):S406–13.

Bernstein JA. Otitis media in children. N Engl J Med. 1995;333(17):1151–2.

Bernstein JA. Pharmacoeconomic considerations for allergen immunotherapy. Clin Allergy Immunol. 2004;18:151–64.

Bernstein JA. Characterizing rhinitis subtypes. Am J Rhinol Allergy. 2013;27(6):457–60.

Bernstein JA, Fox RW, Martin VT, Lockey RF. Headache and facial pain: differential diagnosis and treatment. J Allergy Clin Immunol Pract. 2013;1(3):242–51.

Bernstein JA, Bernstein JS, Makol R, Ward S. Allergic rhinitis: a review. JAMA. 2024; 331(10):866–77.

Casciano J, Krishnan JA, Small MB, Buck PO, Gopalan G, Li C, et al. Value of peripheral blood eosinophil markers to predict severity of asthma. BMC Pulm Med. 2016;16(1):109.

Chitsuthipakorn W, Hoang MP, Kanjanawasee D, Seresirikachorn K, Snidvongs K. Combined medical therapy in the treatment of allergic rhinitis: systematic review and meta-analyses. Int Forum Allergy Rhinol. 2022;12(12):1480–502.

Cho SH, Nanda A, Keswani A, Adinoff A, Baroody FM, Bernstein JA, et al. Nasal allergen challenge (NAC): practical aspects and applications from an EU/US perspective-a work group report of the AAAAI rhinitis, rhinosinusitis and ocular allergy committee. J Allergy Clin Immunol. 2023;151(5):1215–22.

Corren J. The relationship between allergic rhinitis and bronchial asthma. Curr Opin Pulm Med. 1999;5(1):35–7.

Cox L. The role of allergen immunotherapy in the management of allergic rhinitis. Am J Rhinol Allergy. 2016;30:48–53.

Derebery J, Meltzer E, Nathan RA, Stang PE, Campbell UB, Corrao M, et al. Rhinitis symptoms and comorbidities in the United States: burden of rhinitis in America survey. Otolaryngol Head Neck Surg. 2008;139(2):198–205.

Dhamija Y, Epstein TEG, Bernstein DI. Systemic allergic reactions and anaphylaxis associated with allergen immunotherapy. Immunol Allergy Clin N Am. 2022;42(1):105–19.

Dhulipalla S. Ragweed sublingual immunotherapy (SLIT) tablets in allergic rhinoconjunctivitis: a systematic review and meta-analysis. Eur Arch Otorrinolaringol. 2022;279(6):2765–75.
Donald K, Finlay BB. Early-life interactions between the microbiota and immune system: impact on immune system development and atopic disease. Nat Rev Immunol. 2023;
Drazdauskaite G, Layhadi JA, Shamji MH. Mechanisms of allergen immunotherapy in allergic rhinitis. Curr Allergy Asthma Rep. 2020;21(1):2.
Dykewicz MS, Wallace DV, Amrol DJ, Baroody FM, Bernstein JA, Craig TJ, et al. Rhinitis 2020: a practice parameter update. J Allergy Clin Immunol. 2020;146(4):721–67.
Eggleston PA, Butz A, Rand C, Curtin-Brosnan J, Kanchanaraksa S, Swartz L, et al. Home environmental intervention in inner-city asthma: a randomized controlled clinical trial. Ann Allergy Asthma Immunol. 2005;95(6):518–24.
Farraia M, Paciencia I, Castro Mendes F, Cavaleiro Rufo J, Shamji M, Agache I, et al. Allergen immunotherapy for asthma prevention: a systematic review and meta-analysis of randomized and non-randomized controlled studies. Allergy. 2022;77(6):1719–35.
Gergen PJ, Mortimer KM, Eggleston PA, Rosenstreich D, Mitchell H, Ownby D, et al. Results of the National Cooperative Inner-City Asthma Study (NCICAS) environmental intervention to reduce cockroach allergen exposure in inner-city homes. J Allergy Clin Immunol. 1999;103(3 Pt 1):501–6.
Greiner AN, Hellings PW, Rotiroti G, Scadding GK. Allergic rhinitis. Lancet. 2011;378(9809):2112–22.
Greiwe JC, Bernstein JA. Allergic and mixed rhinitis: diagnosis and natural evolution. J Clin Med. 2019;8(11)
Greiwe J, Bernstein JA. Accelerated/rush allergen immunotherapy. Allergy Asthma Proc. 2022;43(4):344–9.
Head K, Snidvongs K, Glew S, Scadding G, Schilder AG, Philpott C, et al. Saline irrigation for allergic rhinitis. Cochrane Database Syst Rev. 2018;6(6):CD012597.
Health Quality Ontario. Skin testing for allergic rhinitis: a health technology assessment; 2016. Available from: http://www.hqontario.ca/Evidence-to-Improve-Care/Journal-Ontario-Health-TechnologyAssessment-Series/rhinitis-testing
Krishnamoorthy M, Mohd Noor N, Mat Lazim N, Abdullah B. Efficacy of Montelukast in allergic rhinitis treatment: a systematic review and meta-analysis. Drugs. 2020;80(17):1831–51.
Kucuksezer UC, Ozdemir C, Yazici D, Pat Y, Mitamura Y, Li M, et al. The epithelial barrier theory: development and exacerbation of allergic and other chronic inflammatory diseases. Asia Pac Allergy. 2023;13(1):28–39.
LeBlanc GDMaSB. Middleton's allergy. 9th ed. Elsevier; 2020.
Lugogo N, Chipps BE, Panettieri RA Jr, Trudo F, Ambrose CS. Long-term use of maintenance systemic corticosteroids is associated with multiple adverse conditions in a large, real-world cohort of US adults with severe asthma. J Asthma Allergy. 2022;15:1753–61.
Martin VT, Taylor F, Gebhardt B, Tomaszewski M, Ellison JS, Martin GV, et al. Allergy and immunotherapy: are they related to migraine headache? Headache. 2011;51(1):8–20.
Martin VT, Fanning KM, Serrano D, Buse DC, Reed ML, Bernstein JA, et al. Chronic rhinitis and its association with headache frequency and disability in persons with migraine: results of the American migraine prevalence and prevention (AMPP) study. Cephalalgia. 2014;34(5):336–48.
Meltzer EO, Nathan R, Derebery J, Stang PE, Campbell UB, Yeh WS, et al. Sleep, quality of life, and productivity impact of nasal symptoms in the United States: findings from the burden of rhinitis in America survey. Allergy Asthma Proc. 2009a;30(3):244–54.
Meltzer EO, Blaiss MS, Derebery MJ, Mahr TA, Gordon BR, Sheth KK, et al. Burden of allergic rhinitis: results from the pediatric allergies in America survey. J Allergy Clin Immunol. 2009b;124(3 Suppl):S43–70.
Meltzer EO, Blaiss MS, Naclerio RM, Stoloff SW, Derebery MJ, Nelson HS, et al. Burden of allergic rhinitis: allergies in America, Latin America, and Asia-Pacific adult surveys. Allergy Asthma Proc. 2012;33(Suppl 1):S113–41.

Meltzer EO, Farrar JR, Sennett C. Findings from an online survey assessing the burden and Management of Seasonal Allergic Rhinoconjunctivitis in US patients. J Allergy Clin Immunol Pract. 2017;5(3):779–89 e6.

Mortada MM, Kurowski M. Challenges in local allergic rhinitis diagnosis, management, and research: current concepts and future perspectives. Medicina. 2023;59(5):929.

Mygind N, Laursen LC, Dahl M. Systemic corticosteroid treatment for seasonal allergic rhinitis: a common but poorly documented therapy. Allergy. 2000;55(1):11–5.

Nguyen DK, Liang J, Durr M. Topical nasal treatment efficacy on adult obstructive sleep apnea severity: a systematic review and meta-analysis. Int Forum Allergy Rhinol. 2021;11(2):153–61.

Okano M, Fujieda S, Gotoh M, Kurono Y, Matsubara A, Ohta N, et al. Executive summary: Japanese guidelines for allergic rhinitis 2020. Allergol Int. 2023;72(1):41–53.

Ozdoganoglu T, Songu M. The burden of allergic rhinitis and asthma. Ther Adv Respir Dis. 2012;6(1):11–23.

Pawankar R, Mori S, Ozu C, Kimura S. Overview on the pathomechanisms of allergic rhinitis. Asia Pac Allergy. 2011;1(3):157–67.

Penagos M, Durham SR. Allergen immunotherapy for long-term tolerance and prevention. J Allergy Clin Immunol. 2022;149(3):802–11.

Rao D, Phipatanakul W. Impact of environmental controls on childhood asthma. Curr Allergy Asthma Rep. 2011;11(5):414–20.

Roland LT, Wise SK, Wang H, Zhang P, Mehta C, Levy JM. The cost of rhinitis in the United States: a national insurance claims analysis. Int Forum Allergy Rhinol. 2021 May;11(5):946–8.

Schwab AD, Poole JA. Mechanistic and therapeutic approaches to occupational exposure-associated allergic and non-allergic asthmatic disease. Curr Allergy Asthma Rep. 2023;23(6):313–24.

Shao Z, Bernstein JA. Occupational rhinitis: classification, diagnosis, and therapeutics. Curr Allergy Asthma Rep. 2019;19(12):54.

Soe KK, Krikeerati T, Pheerapanyawaranun C, Niyomnaitham S, Phinyo P, Thongngarm T. Comparative efficacy and acceptability of licensed dose intranasal corticosteroids for moderate-to-severe allergic rhinitis: a systematic review and network meta-analysis. Front Pharmacol. 2023;14:1184552.

Ulusoy S, Bayar Muluk N, Scadding GK, Passali GS, Dilber M, Gevaert P, et al. The intranasal trigeminal system: roles in rhinitis (allergic and non-allergic). Eur Rev Med Pharmacol Sci. 2022;26(2 Suppl):25–37.

Wimalasena NN, Chang-Richards A, Wang KI, Dirks KN. Housing risk factors associated with respiratory disease: a systematic review. Int J Environ Res Public Health. 2021;18(6)

Zhang R, Zhang L, Li P, Pang K, Liu H, Tian L. Epithelial barrier in the nasal mucosa, related risk factors and diseases. Int Arch Allergy Immunol. 2023;184(5):481–501.

Part II
Prevention and Management

Chapter 4
Preventive Measures for Allergic Rhinitis

Massoud Mahmoudi

Introduction

Management of chronic conditions involves preventive measures and treatment to alleviate the intensity of the recurrences. Based on the type of a disease, the approaches to preventions are different. The strategy to prevent and or reduce the strength of recurring symptoms should be multifactorial. In allergic rhinitis the type of allergens, the place of exposure, the type of habitation, occupation, and the life style are essential factors in implementing a guide for prevention.

Allergens

There are two types of allergens, indoor and outdoor. The outdoor allergens can find their ways to indoor environment through open doors and windows and stay or settle in different types of habitats. The allergic symptoms are set off by exposure to allergens. The type of allergens, the duration and frequency of exposures are keys to formulate plans and recommendations to establish preventive measures for management of allergic rhinitis (Table 4.1).

M. Mahmoudi (✉)
Department of Medicine, University of California San Francisco, San Francisco, CA, USA

American Osteopathic College of Allergy and Immunology, Fountain Hills, AZ, USA

M. Mahmoudi (ed.), *Treatment and Management of Allergic Rhinitis*,
https://doi.org/10.1007/978-3-031-88107-7_4

Table 4.1 Examples of outdoor and indoor allergens

Allergen	Examples
Outdoor allergens	
Tree pollens	Juniper, Cypress, Cedar
Grass pollens	Timothy, Johnson, Rye
Weed pollens	Ragweed, Pigweed
Indoor allergens	
Pets	Cat, dog
Molds	*Aspergilus, penicillium, Cladosporium*
Cockroaches	German cockroach
Dust mites	*Dermatophagoides farinae;* *Dermatophagoides peterossinus*

An Interview With the Allergic Patient

Before guiding the allergic patients by helping them to implement preventive measures in reducing allergen exposure, it is important to know more about them, where they live, and where they work. The following are outlines of pertinent questions in each category:

More About the Allergic Patient

- Are you currently working? Do you go to school?
- Where do you work? In an office building? A factory? A warehouse? A farm? A garden?
- What type of work do you do? Administration? Farming? painting? Warehouse duties? Gardening?
- Is your work or school area dusty?
- Are you exposed to any chemicals at work?
- Any pets in your work or school?

Inquiry of an Outdoor Environment

- Where do you live? In an urban area, Suburban, farm, rural?
- If you live an urban area, do you live by a freeway?
- Is your home in a flat surface? Do live on a hill?
- How is the motor vehicle traffic around your home?
- How is the weather environment around your residence? Hot, cold, windy, rainy?

Inquiry of an Indoor Building, Work or School

- What is the type of building? A single unit, a multilevel building?
- Is there a basement?
- How old is the building?
- What part of the building do you stay and work? Basement, top floor?
- Are there any windows in the work area? If so, are they functional, i.e. can be opened?
- Any history of flooding?
- Any obvious stained walls?
- Are there any plants indoor?
- Anyone bring to work? If not, do you work close to someone who has pet at home?
- How is the indoor environment? Temperature, humidity?
- Are you able to control temperature and humidity in your work area or is it centrally controlled?

Inquiry of an Indoor Home Environment

- Where do you live? An apartment, a house, in a single room? mobile home?
- How old is the building? If old, has it been renovated?
- Do you have a basement? If yes, any history of flooding?
- Any of the walls are stained?
- Do you have a central heating system? If not, how do you heat up the place? With a furnace? An electric portable unit?
- Do you have a central air-conditioning? If not, how do you cool the place? With a fan? An electric portable air-conditioning? A water cooler?
- What type of flooring do you have? Hardwood, linoleum, tile, or carpet? How old are they? have they been changed recently?
- How do you block he sun to the home? Do you have fabric curtains? blinds?
- What type of furniture do you have? leathers? Upholstered material?
- What type of bedding do you have? anything item with feather?
- How often you wash your beddings? What temperature do you use for washing?
- How is the indoor temperature? Do you measure temperature?
- How is he humidity in your place? Do you measure humidity?
- Do you have pets? A cat, a dog, a hamster, a bird? Is there a designated area for your pets or they can move around freely? Do you let your pets to come in your bedrooms?
- Do you have plant at home?
- How you clean your home?
- How often do clean your home?

Outdoor Allergens

Pollens During pollinating season wind scatters pollens in the air. As we go outdoor and inhale the aerosolized pollens, they get into our airway passages and trigger our immune system.

Indoor Allergens

In an indoor environment, we are exposed to various allergens including dust mites, molds, pets, and cockroaches.

The Following Are Common Outdoor Allergens

Pollen

The outdoor pollens include trees, grasses, and weeds. The pollinating season are different for each type of pollen. Familiarity of regional pollination season helps to identify timing for prevention and management of symptoms.

Tree Pollen

Trees usually pollinate during spring. As the climate varies in different regions of the United States and the world, the timing of pollinating season are different.

Grass Pollen

Grasses usually pollinating during summer. As the tree pollens, the timing of pollination varies from one region to another.

Weed Pollen

Weeds usually pollinate during fall. Some weeds grow in a specific region and some grow nationwide, i.e. they can grow in different environments.

Outdoor Measures

The following measures can reduce the allergen exposures:

- Wearing a face mask. Wearing a face mask during days with high pollen counts helps to prevent the upper airways from direct exposure to aerosolized pollens.
- Walking along the lawns/parks. During allergy season, avoid walking along lawns/parks specially when the lawn are freshly cut.
- Close windows during windy and pollinating season to avoid exposure to pollens.
- Do not mow lawns. If you have to, wear a face mask and change the clothing and shower when done.

The Following Are Common Indoor Allergens

Dust Mites

Dust mites are the most common indoor allergens. They are 8-legged. Sightless, arthropods from the family pyroglyphidae. Dusts in crude forms may or may not harbor dust mites. Regardless, it is not possible to differentiate either type with the naked eyes. Two common house dust mites are from genus Dermatophagoides, namely *Dermatophagoides farinae* and *Dermatophagoides peteroyssinus*.

Preventing Measures to Reduce Dust Mites Exposure

Cleaning

General Environment

House dusts are dispersed in most parts of a home. They mostly reside in furnished part of the building like the bedrooms, living rooms, and less in a kitchen. The bathrooms and rest rooms, and garages are not the desired environments for dust mites; of course it also depends on how much of clothing and furniture are placed in those places. The following are some examples of cleaning strategies:

- Remove the unwanted furniture's form the living rooms. This leaves less place for the dusts to settle in.
- Change all upholstered furniture to non-upholstered furniture such as leather or vinyl-like materials. If this is not possible or practical, cover the furniture with dust mite-proof covers when unused.

- Use a damp fabric to wipe the surfaces such as tables, desks, bookshelves, and blinds. More detailed cleaning includes wiping out blades of fans, each object on the tables or shelves one by one as the dusts settles on all objects.
- Vacuuming carpet floors regularly with vacuum with HEPA filtration.
- Cautions about using Acaricdes. These are chemicals that kill mites. They are applied to places where the mites reside and live such as upholstered furniture, bedding, carpets, or fabric curtains. By using these chemicals, we are exposing ourselves specially the younger children to these reagents. Two areas of concerns are safety issue and questionable effectiveness of theses reagents. As such, the use of these chemicals in home are not recommended. In addition, application of Tannic acid, a protein-denaturing agents to carpers in reducing dust mite allergens is not recommended. This is due to its limited effectiveness.
- Hardwood and tiles floors are easier to clean than carpers. If practical, removing of all carpet floors helps to reduce an important dust mites' reservoir.

Bedrooms

The two target areas in controlling dust mites in bedrooms are the floors and beddings. Of course adding furniture in the bedrooms increasing the dust mites population. The following are some control measures for reducing dust mite exposure.

- Encasing pillow cases with dust mite proof encasing prevents the passages of dust mites.
- Avoid using feather pillows as dust mites can live and survive in feathers.
- Avoid using feather comforters.
- Encase mattress and box springs to avoid passages of the dust mites.
- Washing bed sheets and pillowcases with hot water every 1–2 weeks. This is a way to get rid of dust mites. When using hot water, it is recommended to use temperature below 120 degree Fahrenheit to avoid burning skin.

Humidity

- Reducing humidity below 50% is the best intervention to reduce house dust mites. Using a hygrometer helps to keep an eye on the indoor humidity.
- Use a Dehumidifier to reduce the indoor humidity.
- Educating patients about humidifier and dehumidifier as some patients unaware of their dust mite allergies, mistakenly purchase humidifier which leads to worsening of their symptoms.

HEPA Filtration

Use of HEPA filtration alone has limited effectiveness. It all depends on where to place it in the home as the locations of aerosolized dust mites varies in different parts of the home.

Pets

The common pets are cats and dogs. However, many small or large animals are kept as pets. Familiarity with own pets, such as places they like to eat, sleep, or deposit excretes are essential to formulate an effective way to prevent allergic symptoms. As each type of pets carry and express their allergens differently, knowledge of pet allergens are important as we assign a place for our pets in a home. The decision as where we allow the pets to stay affects our level of exposure to the pets and the intensity of allergic symptoms. For example, some keep cats in outdoor environment and others let the cats in the building and even in the bedrooms. Of course by close exposure to pets we increase the chance of expression of the allergy symptoms. The following are common measures to prevent and or reduce allergy symptoms due to pet exposures:

- Keep pets outdoor if possible; this limits the close exposure and prevent or reduce the allergy symptoms.
- If you keep pets in the building, do not let them in the bedroom. Cats and dogs shed hair and by that spread the allergens all over the building.
- Removing the carpers if possible; if not, vacuuming the floor regularly is a way to remove the pet hair.
- Keep smaller pets such as a birds in a cage.
- If you keep a fish in an aquarium, clean the surface of the aquarium to prevent settling of molds
- Washing pets regularly helps to remove some allergens.

Rodents

The common rodents are mouse and rat. They can choose any type of building to reside, a house, a restaurant, a school, or any place they can get access to food to survive. The following are common measures to prevent and or reduce allergy symptoms due to rodents exposures:

- When relocating to a different home to live or a business to work, inspect the building for rodents or sign of rodents in the facility.

- Identify the source of rodents' entrance to the buildings and close it properly to prevent further migration.
- Clean all the food scraps from the building specifically kitchen and the dining room.
- Place mouse and rat traps in areas with high rodent infestation.
- Use rodenticides if fail the other preventive measures.

Cockroaches

- Inspect the building for cockroaches.
- Inspect the area of infestation to see whether able to locate the port of entrance.
- Avoid spilling water and dropping food scrapes in dining area and kitchen.
- use cockroach traps in area of heavy infestation.
- Hire professional exterminator for controlling cockroach population.

Molds

Molds are opportunistic organisms which in right environment can grow in abundance. They grow on damp and moist surface. The common areas are shower curtains, around aquariums, and any accessible wet surfaces. The common indoor molds are *aspergillus, penicillium,* and *Cladosporium.* The following are common measured to prevent mold growth and to remove them from the infected environment.

- Inspect the building for obvious mold growth with special attention to bathrooms, restrooms, and kitchen.
- Look for any leaky faucets or damaged pipes. Repair and repair the defective parts.
- Some contaminated objects can be replaced such as shower curtains. If possible remove the certain and replace them with mildew resistant shower curtain.
- Keep the surface areas dry: kitchen tables, sinks, bathrooms.
- Use bleach to kill mold on surface and then clean are area.
- Ventilate the home: kitchen, bathrooms, basements.

Suggested Reading

Mahmoudi M, editor. Allergy and asthma; practical diagnosis and management. New York: Springer; 2016.

Mahmoudi M. Absolute allergy and immunology board review. New York: Springer; 2022.

Mahmoudi M. Allergy and asthma made ridiculously simple. 2nd ed. Florida: MedMaster; 2025.

Mahmoudi M, Ledford D, Craig T, editors. Allergy and asthma, the basics, to best practices. New York: Springer; 2019.

Phipatanakul W, Matsui E, Portnoy, ad J.E.Ad. Environmental assessment and exposure reduction for rodents: a practice parameter. Ann Allergy Asthma Immunol. 2012;109:375–8.

Portnoy J, Kennedy J, Sublett J. Environmental assessment and exposure control: a practice parameter-furry animals. Ann Allergy Asthma Immunol. 2012;108:223.

Portnoy J, et al. Environmental assessment and exposure reduction of cockroaches: a practice parameter. J Allergy Clin Immunol. 2013;132(4):802–8.

Chapter 5
Oral Medications in Treatment of Allergic Rhinitis

Gisoo Ghaffari and Shane Stone

Introduction

Allergic rhinitis (AR) is a prevalent condition in the United States that significantly impacts quality of life. It is characterized by symptoms such as rhinorrhea, nasal congestion, sneezing, and nasal itching, which can lead to fatigue, irritability, depression, sleep disturbances, and hindered physical and social functioning. These symptoms often result in absenteeism from work and school, as well as decreased work productivity, imposing a substantial economic burden on society. Managing AR involves various strategies, including allergen avoidance, symptomatic relief through medications, and disease modification via allergen immunotherapy. Oral medications, particularly those aimed at alleviating symptoms, are crucial in AR management and can also be useful to address associated symptoms affecting the eyes, ears, and throat.

Rhinitis is generally categorized into allergic and nonallergic types based on the underlying pathogenic mechanism. However, it's essential to distinguish it from other conditions that share similar symptoms. Allergic rhinitis involves Immunoglobulin E (IgE)-mediated inflammation of the nasal mucosa, while non-allergic rhinitis (NAR) is characterized by mechanisms independent of IgE. NAR encompasses various subtypes, including vasomotor, infectious, food-induced, hormonal, drug-induced, nonallergic occupational, atrophic, NAR with eosinophilia

G. Ghaffari (✉)
Division of Pulmonary, Allergy and Critical Care Medicine, Pennsylvania State College of Medicine, Hershey, PA, USA
e-mail: gghaffari@pennstatehealth.psu.edu

S. Stone
Department of Internal Medicine-Pediatrics, Pennsylvania State College of Medicine, Hershey, PA, USA
e-mail: sstone1@pennstatehealth.psu.edu

M. Mahmoudi (ed.), *Treatment and Management of Allergic Rhinitis*,
https://doi.org/10.1007/978-3-031-88107-7_5

syndrome (NARES), and rhinitis of the elderly. Additionally, several other conditions present overlapping symptoms with rhinitis, such as rhinosinusitis with and without nasal polyps, cerebrospinal fluid rhinorrhea, ciliary dyskinesia syndrome, and structural/mechanical factors, such as congenital anomalies, deviated septum, and pharyngo-nasal reflux (Dykewicz et al. 2020).

The foundational step in diagnosing allergic rhinitis involves obtaining a thorough clinical history. Essential details such as age of onset, duration, frequency, and severity of symptoms should be carefully assessed, alongside identification of triggers and seasonal patterns. Allergic rhinitis predominantly affects younger individuals with a familial predisposition to atopy and often displays clear seasonal changes or environmental triggers. Common symptoms of AR include watery rhinorrhea, sneezing, and nasal itching, while non-allergic rhinitis (NAR) tends to manifest with pronounced nasal congestion and mucoid rhinorrhea, with sneezing and pruritus being less prevalent. Additionally, allergic rhinitis frequently presents with extra nasal symptoms such as ocular pruritis, watery red eyes, sore throat, chronic cough, and eustachian tube dysfunction. Distinguishing these differences is crucial as treatment approaches can differ between AR, NAR, and other similar conditions. For instance, while oral antihistamines are considered a first-line therapy for allergic rhinitis, they have no proven efficacy for non-allergic rhinitis (Dykewicz et al. 2020).

The management of AR is further guided by disease classification based on the frequency and severity of symptoms. Traditionally, AR was categorized into seasonal and perennial variants. However, this classification system had limitations, leading to the adoption of more recent guidelines that classify AR as either intermittent or persistent, and as mild or moderate/severe. Treatment recommendations vary based on this classification. For instance, oral therapies are typically considered first-line for intermittent symptoms whereas moderate/severe and persistent symptoms often necessitate additional targeted intranasal therapies (Dykewicz et al. 2020). Treatment decisions are also guided by factors such as drug-specific considerations including efficacy, time to onset, dosing frequency, tolerability, and patient preference for monotherapy. For instance, patients may prefer oral therapies over intranasal medications due to concerns about taste, nasal dryness, and nosebleeds. Providers may also opt for oral medications to help address extra-nasal symptoms like cough and conjunctivitis or in cases of severe nasal obstruction where intranasal drug delivery is hindered.

In this chapter, we will delve into the various oral medications commonly utilized in the treatment of AR, including conventional treatments with oral antihistamines, leukotriene receptor antagonists, oral decongestants, and corticosteroids. Additionally, we will discuss alternative therapies with less established evidence but potential efficacy in AR management, such as probiotics, vitamin supplements, honey, and herbal medicines (Table 5.1). Each medication will be examined in terms of its unique mechanism of action and specific indications within the context of AR treatment (Table 5.2).

Table 5.1 Summary of evidence and recommendations for oral medications in the treatment of AR

Conventional therapies			
Antihistamines	**LTRA**	**Corticosteroids**	**Decongestants**
Second generation OAHs are recommended as a 1st line option for treatment of mild and moderate/severe intermittent AR as well as mild persistent AR. First generation OAH are recommended *against* due to increased risk for adverse effects.	LTRA are modestly effective in the treatment of AR and provide particular benefit in patients with comorbid asthma. LTRA should *not* be selected as the initial agent for treatment of AR due to their risk of neuropsychiatric events.	A short course (5–7 days) of oral steroids may be considered for the treatment of very severe or intractable AR. Depot parenteral corticosteroids are recommended *against* due to the potential risk of systemic side effects.	Oral decongestants can be used for short term symptom relief in the management of AR. Caution should be used in older adults, children < 4 years old, and in patients with certain predisposing conditions. Avoid during the 1st trimester of pregnancy due to risk of birth defects.
Non-conventional therapies			
Probiotics	Vitamins	Honey	Chinese herbal medicine (CHM)
Probiotics may play a protective role in the prevention of atopic conditions through down-regulation of Th2 pathways. There is mixed evidence to support the use of probiotics, but they can be considered as an adjuvant treatment for AR due to their tolerability and minimal side effect profile.	Vitamin A and C have no impact on outcomes in AR. Vitamin E deficiency has been associated with AR, but there is no consistent improvement in symptoms with vitamin E supplementation. Vitamin D supplementation has no benefits in adults but may improve symptoms associated with AR in children.	There is no evidence to support the use of honey in the treatment of AR. Honey is a natural cough suppressant that may play a role in the management of cough associated with postnasal drip in AR.	Many herbal medications have been shown to have immunomodulatory effects. CHM shows a slight trend toward benefit in treatment of AR but support for their use is limited by poor study quality. Some herbal preparations contain toxic chemicals, like pyrrolizidine alkaloids, that can cause harm.

Table 5.2 Response of each symptom of allergic rhino-conjunctivitis to various medications

Agent	Sneezing	Itching	Congestion	Rhinorrhea	Eye symptoms
Oral antihistamines	++	++	+/–	++	++
Nasal antihistamines	+	+	+	+	–
Intranasal corticosteroids	++	++	+++	++	+
Leukotriene modifiers	+	+	+	+	+
Oral decongestants	–	–	++	–	–
Nasal decongestants	–	–	+++	–	–
Nasal mast-cell stabilizers	+	+	+	+	–

+: mild response; ++: moderate response; +++: robust response; +/– : mild/no response

Oral Antihistamines

Oral antihistamines are a class of medications used to treat a range of histamine-mediated conditions. These drugs can be categorized into two classes: those targeting the H1 receptor and those targeting the H2 receptor. Of these, H1-antihistamines hold particular significance in managing allergic conditions, given histamine's central role in IgE-mediated reactions. In this section, we will examine clinically relevant information about histamine and the H1 receptor, alongside key considerations for selecting and monitoring antihistamines in the context of allergic rhinitis.

Histamine: Histamine is a chemical mediator that plays a vital role in human health. It exerts its influence through specific receptors that are classified into four subtypes: H1 through H4. Activation of the H1 receptor, specifically, contributes to numerous physiological processes, including cell proliferation and differentiation, embryonic development, hematopoiesis, wound healing, endocrine homeostasis, and neurotransmission within the central nervous system. Moreover, the H1 receptor plays a pivotal role in the intricate system of inflammation and immune regulation whereby it amplifies the release of mast cell mediators and enhances antigen-presenting cell capacity. Additionally, it downregulates humoral immunity while fostering T-helper 1 proliferation, Interferon-γ production, cellular adhesion molecule expression, and the chemotaxis of eosinophils and neutrophils (Simons and Simons 2011).

Histamine receptor: Histamine exerts its effects through membrane-bound G-protein coupled receptors, which are widely distributed throughout the body. They are particularly prevalent in the smooth muscle of the bronchi, gastrointestinal tract, uterus, large blood vessels, and the central nervous system. These receptors exhibit constitutive activity and can be conceptualized as a group of "cellular switches" existing in equilibrium between the active or "on" state and the inactive or "off" state. In the presence of histamine, the receptor stabilizes in its active conformation, shifting the equilibrium to the "on" position. Conversely, in the presence of H1-antihistamines, which are structurally unrelated to histamine and bind to a different site on the receptor, the receptor stabilizes in the inactive conformation and swings the equilibrium towards the "off" position. Because of this, antihistamines are considered inverse agonists rather than receptor antagonists, in that they produce the opposite effect of histamine on the receptor (Simons and Simons 2011).

H1-antihistamines: In allergic rhinitis, histamine binding to H1 receptors triggers vasodilation, increased vascular permeability, smooth muscle contraction, and edema in the nasal mucosa, contributing to hallmark symptoms such as rhinorrhea, sneezing, nasal itching, and congestion. H1-antihistamines directly mitigate allergic inflammation by impeding histamine's actions at H1 receptors on sensory neurons and small blood vessels. They also diminish antigen presentation, chemotaxis, and the expression of proinflammatory cytokines and cell adhesion molecules by suppressing the ubiquitous transcription factor nuclear factor-κB. Moreover, at elevated concentrations, H1-antihistamines have demonstrated inhibition of mast cell activation and histamine release (Simons and Simons 2011).

H1-antihistamines represent the largest class of medications prescribed for the treatment of allergic conditions. They are typically categorized into two groups based on their activity in the central nervous system (CNS). They are also differentiated by their specificity for histamine receptors and associated side effect profiles. First-generation antihistamines, characterized by their lipophilic nature, easily traverse the blood-brain barrier (BBB) and inhibit histaminergic neurotransmission within the CNS, whereas second-generation antihistamines exhibit minimal BBB penetration. Consequently, the first-generation drugs are more prone to CNS-related adverse effects such as sedation, drowsiness, fatigue, and impaired cognitive function, learning, and memory. Moreover, they demonstrate poor selectivity for the H1 receptor and have antagonistic effects on central and peripheral muscarinic, serotonergic, and alpha-1 adrenergic receptors, leading to various adverse effects including mydriasis, dry eyes, dry mouth, constipation, urinary retention, increased appetite, weight gain, dizziness, and orthostatic hypotension. In contrast, second-generation H1-antihistamines are largely devoid of central nervous system (CNS) side effects and do not interact with muscarinic, serotonergic, or alpha-adrenergic receptors, making them the preferred drug of choice for the treatment of allergic rhinitis (Simons and Simons 2011).

Oral second-generation H1-antihistamines have strong evidence supporting their efficacy. They are effective in preventing and alleviating the early allergic response that leads to sneezing, itching, and rhinorrhea. Additionally, they may offer a small benefit in relief of nasal congestion associated with the late allergic response. Compared to other agents, they exhibit superior efficacy to mast cell stabilizers and leukotriene receptor antagonists, though they are less effective than nasal glucocorticoids. In clinical practice, oral second-generation H1-antihistamines are recommended as a first-line treatment for mild to moderate/severe intermittent allergic rhinitis as well as for mild persistent allergic rhinitis. Notably, they have little to no role in the treatment of non-allergic rhinitis (Dykewicz et al. 2020).

When choosing an oral antihistamine for allergic rhinitis, it's essential to adopt a patient-centered approach. This involves considering the efficacy and potential side effects of each antihistamine while taking in-to account individual preferences and tolerances. Factors such as sedation and impact on daily activities, lifestyle, adherence to treatment, concurrent medical conditions, cost, pregnancy and breastfeeding status, and other medications being taken should all be weighed. Research from various large trials and meta-analyses indicates that all second-generation antihistamines are effective in alleviating allergic rhinitis symptoms, with similar overall efficacy. However, there are differences in onset of action, duration of effect, and side effect profiles among these agents. For example, both desloratadine and fexofenadine significantly reduce total symptom scores and nasal symptoms, with fexofenadine showing no significant adverse effects compared to placebo (Linton et al. 2023). Fexofenadine is preferred for occupations requiring optimal alertness, memory, and cognition due to its minimal crossing of the blood-brain barrier. However, its shorter duration of action necessitates twice-daily dosing, which may pose challenges for some patients in terms of medication adherence. Levocetirizine, though mildly sedating, has fewer sedative effects compared to first-generation antihistamines and outperforms loratadine in improving total symptom scores. Cetirizine, while classified as sedating, particularly in children, is well tolerated and remains widely used. Newer agents like bilastine and rupatadine also show promise. Bilastine offers efficacy comparable to cetirizine and fexofenadine but with fewer instances of somnolence and fatigue. Rupatadine demonstrates a favorable risk-benefit profile in allergic rhinitis treatment (Linton et al. 2023).

While second-generation antihistamines are generally well tolerated, it's important to review common side effects. These may include fatigue, dizziness, dry mouth, and gastrointestinal disturbances. Notably, concerns were raised regarding potential cardiotoxicity with the initial two second-generation antihistamines—terfenadine and astemizole. These medications were associated with QT interval prolongation and the development of torsades de pointes. However, multiple studies have confirmed that presently available second-generation antihistamines do not elicit these effects, even when administered at doses several times higher than the recommended doses. This indicates that the likelihood of inducing ventricular arrhythmias is not a class-effect shared among all second-generation antihistamines (DuBuske 1999). Table 5.3 summarizes the features of various second-generation, long-acting antihistaminic agents. (Table 5.3).

Table 5.3 Comparison of features of second generation anti-histamines

Second generation antihistamine	Standard dosage for age	Contraindications	Most common side effects	Notes
Loratadine	≥ 2 to 6 years: 5 mg daily ≥6 years: 10 mg daily	Hypersensitivity	Headache, low sedative potential	Safest during the last trimester of pregnancy. Not metabolized by the CYP3A4
Desloratadine	6 to ≤11 months: 1mg daily 1 to ≤5 years: 1.25mg daily 6 to 11 years: 5–10 mg daily ≥12 years: 10 mg daily	Hypersensitivity	Headache, diarrhea, low sedative potential	Sx more potent than loratadine in suppressing wheals. Safest in patients with renal failure.
Cetirizine	6 to <12 months: 2.5 mg daily 1 to <2 years: 2.5 mg once daily 2 to 5 years: 2.5–5 mg daily 6 to 11 years: 5–10 mg daily ≥12 years: 10 mg daily	Hypersensitivity	Drowsiness, headache	Can be used during the last trimester in pregnancy

(continued)

Table 5.3 (continued)

Second generation antihistamine	Standard dosage for age	Contraindications	Most common side effects	Notes
Levocetirizine	> 6 months to <5 years: 1.25 mg daily 6 to 11 years: 2.5 mg daily ≥12 years: 5 mg daily	Hypersensitivity, end stage renal disease, hemodialysis, patients < 11 year with renal impairment	Diarrhea, drowsiness	
Fexofenadine	≥6 months to <2 years: 15 mg twice daily ≥2 to <12 years: 30 mg twice daily ≥12 years: 60 mg twice daily	Hypersensitivity	Headache, vomiting, low sedative potential	Safest in patient with renal failure. Not metabolized by liver/ the CYP3A4. Does not require dose adjustment in mild renal/liver dysfunction
Rupatadine	≥2 to <12 years: 10 kg to 25 kg: 2.5 mg daily ≥25 kg: 5 mg daily > 12 years: 5 mg daily	Hypersensitivity, history of QTc prolongation and/ or torsades de pointes, concurrent use of CYP3A4 inhibitors or other QTc prolonging drugs	Drowsiness/ low sedative potential, headache	
Bilastine	≥12 years: 20 mg daily	Hypersensitivity, history of QTc prolongation and/ or torsades de pointes,	Drowsiness/ low sedative potential, headache	

Leukotriene Receptor Antagonists

Leukotrienes (LT) are inflammatory lipid mediators implicated in numerous allergic conditions. They belong to the eicosanoid family and are synthesized by leukocytes in response to various immunologic and non-immunologic triggers. Serving as key players in the inflammatory cascade, LTs exert their effects by interacting with multiple receptors (Cuzzo and Lappin 2024). Leukotriene receptor antagonists (LTRA) constitute a class of medications that inhibit the actions of these receptors, and thus contribute to the management of allergic rhinitis.

In response to an appropriate stimulus, leukotrienes are synthesized via the 5-lipoxygenase pathway of arachidonic acid metabolism. Arachidonic acid, a fatty acid constituent of cell membranes, is liberated into the cytoplasm by phospholipase A, where it undergoes further modification by 5-lipoxygenase to generate leukotriene A (LTA). LTA serves as a precursor molecule for the synthesis of other leukotrienes, including dihydroxy leukotriene (LTB4) and cysteinyl leukotrienes (LTC4, LTD4, LTE4). The effects of leukotrienes vary; typically, LTB4, synthesized by neutrophils at inflammatory sites, acts as a potent chemoattractant for neutrophils, while cysteinyl leukotrienes, produced by eosinophils, basophils, and mast cells, mediate bronchoconstriction, mucus secretion, vascular permeability, and tissue fibrosis. Additionally, leukotrienes promote leukocyte migration into tissues and enhance the effects of type 2 T helper cells (Duroudier et al. 2009).

In the context of allergic rhinitis, cysteinyl leukotrienes (CysLTs) function as key mediators of nasal allergic inflammation. These molecules contribute to allergic sensitization by augmenting dendritic cell-stimulated antigen presentation and modulate clinical symptoms, particularly sneezing and rhinorrhea, through activation of the CysLTR1 receptor (Duroudier et al. 2009). Leukotriene receptor antagonists (LTRA) represent a class of medications that target the CysLT1 receptor and its downstream effects. Montelukast, zafirlukast, and pranlukast are three LTRA developed and utilized in clinical practice, with montelukast being the sole agent approved for treatment of allergic rhinitis. Alternatively, leukotriene synthesis inhibitors (LTSI) are a class of drugs that impede the formation of all leukotrienes through inhibition of 5-lipoxygenase. Zileuton is the sole drug approved in this category, but its application is limited to asthma maintenance therapy, and it plays no role in allergic rhinitis management.

Montelukast, initially approved in 1998, is a LTRA marketed for the treatment of intermittent allergic rhinitis in adults and children over 2 years of age, as well as persistent allergic rhinitis in adults and children over 6 months of age. Montelukast has shown modest effectiveness in treating AR, with various reviews suggesting its efficacy is similar to oral antihistamines, often comparing it to loratadine; however, other sources find that LTRAs are less effective than antihistamines (Dykewicz et al. 2020). Generally, well tolerated, its side effects are infrequent, with the most common including upper respiratory infection, fever, headache, pharyngitis, cough, abdominal pain, diarrhea, and otitis media. Montelukast has been promoted for its utility as monotherapy in treating allergic rhinitis in individuals with mild persistent asthma due to its steroid-sparing effects and ability to treat both upper and lower allergic airway diseases. However, following post-marketing surveillance, rare drug-induced neuropsychiatric events, such as aggression, depression, and suicidal ideation and behavior, were reported. In March 2020, the US FDA raised safety concerns regarding montelukast and its potential for serious neuropsychiatric events. Consequently, a black box warning, the FDA's most prominent alert, was added to prescribing information. Recent guidelines now advocate for the reserved use of montelukast, specifically recommending it for patients who either do not respond well to or cannot tolerate other allergy medications (Dykewicz et al. 2020).

In clinical practice, combining an LTRA with an oral antihistamine has demonstrated superiority over using either agent alone, showing comparable effectiveness to monotherapy with an intranasal corticosteroid. However, this combined therapy may entail higher costs and increased treatment complexity. As mentioned above, Montelukast has demonstrated benefits in managing both AR and asthma. However, given its potential risks compared to oral antihistamines, clinicians must carefully assess the advantages of montelukast monotherapy in treating AR with concurrent asthma against the option of using an inhaled corticosteroid for asthma alongside an antihistamine or INCS for AR (Dykewicz et al. 2020).

Oral Decongestants

Nasal congestion is a common symptom in various conditions, such as the common cold, rhinosinusitis, nasal polyps, and allergic rhinitis. In AR, nasal congestion primarily results from the infiltration of inflammatory cells during the late allergic response. Congestion is frequently cited as one of the most bothersome symptoms in AR and often remains inadequately treated by conventional medications like oral antihistamines. Additionally, significant edema in the nasal mucosa can prevent the effectiveness of intranasal antihistamines and intranasal corticosteroids by hindering their ability to reach their target. In such scenarios, oral decongestants may be considered for short-term relief of symptoms.

Nasal decongestants, also known simply as decongestants, belong to a class of medications designed to alleviate congestion in the upper respiratory tract. They achieve this effect by stimulating post-junctional alpha-adrenergic receptors, either through direct receptor binding or by augmenting the release of norepinephrine, which induces vasoconstriction. This constriction reduces blood flow through the nasal mucosa, leading to a reduction in tissue size (Johnson and Hricik 1993). Decongestants trace their roots to various species of Ephedra, a seed-producing plant, with Ephedra sinica, commonly known as Ma Huang, being the most prevalent. The historical use of Ephedra in medicine spans millennia, documented in China for over 5000 years and in the Middle East for over 2000 years, where it was utilized for treating conditions such as asthma, colds, hay fever, edema, bronchitis, urticaria, hypotension, and rheumatism. In more recent times, it has also gained popularity as a stimulant for appetite suppression and weight loss, making it sought after by athletes, bodybuilders, and students (Głowacka and Wiela-Hojeńska 2021).

Presently, two oral decongestants are commercially available: pseudoephedrine (PSE) and phenylephrine. Among these, PSE has demonstrated remarkable efficacy in alleviating nasal congestion, whereas research indicates that oral phenylephrine offers no discernible advantage over a placebo, even at doses up to 40 mg. However, pseudoephedrine is a critical component in the illicit production of methamphetamine. Consequently, in the United States, regulations have been enforced to restrict its availability, leading to its substitution with oral phenylephrine in numerous formulations (Dykewicz et al. 2020).

In practice, decongestants are not recommended for routine use in AR but can be considered as a short-term rescue therapy for severe or prolonged symptoms. Additionally, data suggests that combining oral decongestants with oral antihistamines is more effective in mitigating symptoms of AR compared to each component individually. For this purpose, a combination medication containing loratadine/pseudoephedrine is available (Dykewicz et al. 2020).

When used at appropriate doses, oral decongestants are typically well tolerated. Common adverse effects include central nervous system stimulation (anxiety, insomnia, tremors), headache, dizziness, nausea, loss of appetite, and palpitations. While elevated blood pressure has been reported, its true incidence remains controversial. A comprehensive meta-analysis demonstrated that pseudoephedrine (PSE) administered at the recommended dose had no significant impact on blood pressure in healthy individuals or those with controlled hypertension (Głowacka and Wiela-Hojeńska 2021). Rare adverse events, including ischemic colitis, stroke, seizures, and skin reactions, have been documented, alongside reports in infants and young children of agitated psychosis, ataxia, hallucinations, and fatalities. Importantly, decongestants should be avoided during pregnancy due to the heightened risk of gastroschisis, particularly during the first trimester, as highlighted by epidemiological studies indicating an increased risk of various birth defects involving the heart, eyes, ears, gut, abdominal wall, and feet. Given their potential for drug interactions, oral decongestants should also be avoided in patients concurrently taking monoamine oxidase inhibitors and other vasoactive drugs like ergotamine, linezolid, and bromocriptine. Moreover, decongestants should be used with caution in patients with specific medical conditions, including a history of cardiac arrhythmia, angina, cerebrovascular disease, uncontrolled hypertension, bladder outlet obstruction, glaucoma, hyperthyroidism, or Tourette syndrome (Dykewicz et al. 2020).

Oral Corticosteroids

Oral corticosteroids (CS) are a highly effective group of medications known for their ability to reduce inflammation by modulating the immune response. Clinically utilized for decades, they serve as potent anti-inflammatory and immunosuppressive agents and play a role in the management of many allergic conditions. However, their utility in the treatment of allergic rhinitis is limited, owing to their array of systemic side effects.

Oral CS exert their anti-inflammatory effects primarily through gene transcription regulation. Characterized by their lipophobic nature, they passively diffuse across the cell membrane and bind to cytoplasmic glucocorticoid receptors (GR). Upon binding, the steroid-receptor complex trans-locates to the nucleus and binds to specific chromatin sites known as glucocorticoid response elements (GRE), positioned upstream of steroid-responsive genes. This complex interaction leads to the modulation of various genes implicated in inflammation. Specifically, it stimulates the synthesis of anti-inflammatory cytokines, suppresses pro-inflammatory cytokines, and directly interacts with other transcription factors activated during chronic inflammation (Yasir et al. 2024).

From a clinical perspective, corticosteroids exert regulatory control over both the early and late stages of the inflammatory response in allergic rhinitis. During the early phase, they mitigate the hyperresponsiveness of the nasal mucosa to histamine and prevent the heightened sensitivity to allergens following allergen exposure, known as the priming effect. Additionally, corticosteroids attenuate the infiltration of eosinophils and basophils while reducing the production and release of cytokines and chemokines from T lymphocytes, which are hallmark features of the late-phase response (Nelson 1999).

While effective in managing clinical symptoms, oral CS are associated with well-recognized systemic side effects that constrain their utility. This is partly attributed to their diverse mechanisms, encompassing gene transcription regulation, suppression of the hypothalamic-pituitary-adrenal (HPA) axis, mineralocorticoid receptor activation, and modulation of calcium and sodium transport across cell membranes. Common adverse effects linked with oral CS include increased appetite, weight gain, and insomnia. However, more severe complications encompass osteoporosis, adrenal suppression, hyperglycemia, dyslipidemia, cardiovascular disease, Cushing's syndrome, psychiatric disturbances, and immunosuppression, among others. Of the factors influencing the occurrence of adverse effects, dosage and treatment duration are the most influential. When administered at appropriate dosages for limited durations, oral CS generally pose a low risk of harm. However, supratherapeutic doses given over extended periods of time or abrupt cessation can yield catastrophic consequences. Additionally, the route of administration constitutes an important risk factor, with non-systemic or local therapies being preferred for their capacity to mitigate systemic effects (Yasir et al. 2024).

In clinical practice, oral CS have largely been supplanted by intranasal preparations. However, specific circumstances may necessitate systemic steroid use. For instance, in severe or refractory AR cases, clinicians might opt for a brief course (5–7 days) of oral CS. Moreover, patients with significant nasal obstruction impeding intranasal medication delivery or penetration may benefit from oral CS. Nevertheless, it's crucial for clinicians to engage patients in a shared discussion regarding potential risks and benefits, especially among elderly individuals or those with systemic conditions like diabetes, glaucoma, or heart disease. Additionally, some providers may consider depot parenteral corticosteroids an appealing option due to their extended duration of action, capable of addressing an entire allergy season. However, concerns arise regarding the heightened risk of adrenal suppression associated with depot corticosteroids compared to short courses of short-acting corticosteroids. Consequently, current guidelines advise against depot corticosteroid use in AR (Dykewicz et al. 2020).

Probiotics

The microbiome or the community of microorganisms that live in and on our bodies plays an important role in the maintenance of health and well-being. Increasingly, we have learned that disturbances in the microbiome are linked to a broad array of problems. In particular, reduced bacterial diversity in the intestinal flora of infants within the first 6 years of life has been shown to predispose to the development of AR, and maintenance of diversity of the gut and skin microbiome has been associated with protective effects against atopic diseases (Bisgaard et al. 2011), with probiotics supplementation potentially aiding this protection.

Probiotics have been shown to have a modulatory effect on immune function by regulating interactions between dendritic cells, T cells, bacterial metabolites, and cytokines in the gut-associated lymphoid tissue. They also upregulate T-regulatory cells via Interleukin-10 and Transforming Growth Factor TGF-β and downregulate the allergy-associated T-helper 2pathway through suppression of Interleukin-4, total IgE, IgG1, and IgA (Özdemir 2010).

Notwithstanding this, there is mixed evidence to support the clinical use of probiotics in AR. A large meta-analysis found inconsistent benefits of giving probiotics to pregnant mothers or infants for the prevention of various atopic diseases (Lopez-Santamarina et al. 2021), while data from other studies suggest that probiotic supplementation, particularly Lactobacillus and Bifidobacterium spp., has a clear benefit in the reduction of AR-related symptoms in both adults and children (Luo et al. 2022). Interpretation of studies involving probiotics is limited by the heterogeneity of age, diagnosis, interventions, and outcomes, and the variation in organism and dosing across trials, making it difficult to give specific recommendations about treatment. There is also controversy about the potential risk of administering opportunistic bacteria, particularly in children. Nevertheless, probiotics are inexpensive and generally well tolerated with minimal side effects. Therefore, the adjuvant use of probiotics may be considered in patients with AR.

Vitamin Supplementation

Numerous studies have investigated the role of various vitamins in allergic rhinitis. Vitamin A, C, and D have garnered particular attention due to their influence on immune function. These vitamins have been shown to bolster both humoral and cellular immune responses. Notably, vitamin D's immunomodulatory properties are well-documented, affecting T cell activation, cytokine production, and the inhibition of B lymphocytes. Additionally, it plays a crucial role in balancing the Th1/Th2 response and is implicated in the suppression of type 1 inflammatory cytokines (such as interferon-gamma (IFN-γ), interleukins 2, 12, Tumor Necrosis Factor) while enhancing type 2 cytokines (Mitra et al. 2022).

Upon reviewing the available literature, neither vitamin A nor vitamin C levels are associated with allergic rhinitis (AR), nor does their supplementation improve symptoms (García-García et al. 2023). As for vitamin D, numerous clinical and experimental studies have investigated its relationship with AR but have yielded varying and sometimes conflicting results. Clinical investigations suggest a modest inclination towards a correlation between low serum vitamin D levels and the likelihood of AR, particularly among children. However, there is insufficient evidence to support the effectiveness of vitamin D supplementation in preventing AR in pediatric or adult populations. Nonetheless, healthcare providers should consider assessing for vitamin D deficiency when managing AR, especially in children (Kim et al. 2016).

Complementary and Alternative Medicine

The use of complementary or alternative medicine (CAM) is widespread in the world, with common examples including acupuncture, ayurveda, naturopathy and Chinese herbal medicine (CHM). Due to the increasing use of CAM among healthcare consumers, it is important to be aware of these products to provide counseling to patients and discuss potential side effects and drug interactions. Given the focus of this chapter, we will discuss the use of CHM and honey for the treatment of AR.

Herbal medications: For centuries, CHM has been used to treat numerous ailments, including nasal symptoms related to allergies. Many of these products are reported to possess anti-allergic, anti-inflammatory and immunomodulatory effects, such as the inhibition of mast cell mediators, modulation of serum IgE levels, and regulation of lymphocyte and/or macrophage activity, which may be beneficial in the treatment of AR (Xue et al. 2024). In clinical practice, CHM has been shown to have a trend toward benefit when compared to placebo. There also seems to be slight superiority of CHM when used in combination with pharmacotherapy compared to pharmacotherapy alone. It should be noted that most studies that evaluate CHM are small, lack appropriate methodology, and can be difficult to interpret due to differences in product composition. For this reason, professional societies are not able to provide formal recommendations for or against their use (Dykewicz et al. 2020).

Amongst the herbal preparations, several products have been associated with positive outcomes on symptoms scores, but one product in particular, Petasites hybrids (butterbur), has been shown to have the most promising data. In a systematic review, butterbur consistently improved symptoms and QOL comparable to a non-sedating antihistamine, and it received a moderate strength recommendation to support its use in AR. However, more studies are needed to demonstrate its efficacy and safety. Providers should also be aware that many of these preparations can be toxic. For instance, unprocessed butterbur can contain chemicals called pyrrolizidine alkaloids (PAs) that cause damage to the liver, lungs, and endothelium, and have possible associations with cancer. There is also a potential for allergic reactions to butterbur in patients sensitized to ragweed, chrysanthemums, marigolds, and daisies (Dykewicz et al. 2020).

Honey: Honey is a natural substance that is promoted for its many health benefits in naturopathic medicine. Honey contains phytochemical compounds that are reported to have anti-inflammatory, antioxidant, anti-microbial, anti-diabetic, anti-cancer, and cardiovascular disease prevention effects. In relation to allergic rhinitis, "local" honey is commonly recommended as a "natural" treatment due to its content of local pollens and environmental antigens. It is hypothesized that recurrent exposure to these antigens relieves seasonal allergies by improving tolerance similar to allergen immunotherapy (AIT). When studied in vitro, honey has been shown to inhibit mast cell degranulation, anti-allergen IgE levels, and improve histopathological parameters of allergic asthma (Aw Yong et al. 2021). There are, however, several key differences between honey and AIT. With immunotherapy, patients are given small doses of allergens that they are known to be sensitized to, but with honey patients are exposed to random amounts and types of pollen to which they may or may not be allergic. Additionally, pollen contained in honey often comes from the flowers that are encountered by bees but lacks many of the pollens that are responsible for AR, like grass, tree, and weed pollens (Yuko and Cherian 2024). When studied clinically, a small study showed modest improvement in AR symptoms, but participants were required to ingest high daily doses of honey and were on concomitant antihistamine therapy, making the results difficult to interpret (Asha'ari et al. 2013).

Summary

Allergic rhinitis is a common condition that has significant impacts on quality of life. Multiple strategies exist to manage AR, including allergen avoidance, symptom management, and disease modification with allergen immunotherapy. In the treatment framework, oral medications play a large role in the symptomatic treatment of AR, particularly the second-generation antihistamines. As newer treatment options and safety data become available, certain oral medications like oral corticosteroids and leukotriene receptor antagonists have fallen out of favor. However, they still maintain a role in the treatment of AR. Additionally, other therapies like probiotics, vitamin supplements, Chinese herbal medicine, and honey may have mild impacts on symptom control in AR, but the data to fully endorse them is inadequate and more studies are needed to demonstrate their efficacy.

References

Asha'ari ZA, Ahmad MZ, Din WS, Hussin CM, Leman I. Ingestion of honey improves the symptoms of allergic rhinitis: evidence from a randomized placebo-controlled trial in the East Coast of Peninsular Malaysia. Ann Saudi Med. 2013;33(5):469–75.

Aw Yong PY, Islam F, Harith HH, Israf DA, Tan JW, Tham CL. The potential use of honey as a remedy for allergic diseases: a mini review. Front Pharmacol. 2021;11:599080.

Bisgaard H, Li N, Bonnelykke K, Chawes BLK, Skov T, Paludan-Müller G, et al. Reduced diversity of the intestinal microbiota during infancy is associated with increased risk of allergic disease at school age. J Allergy Clin Immunol. 2011;128(3):646–52.

Cuzzo B, Lappin SL. Physiology, leukotrienes. In: StatPearls. Treasure Island (FL): StatPearls Publishing; 2024. Available from: https://www.ncbi.nlm.nih.gov/books/NBK526114/

DuBuske LM. Second-generation antihistamines: the risk of ventricular arrhythmias. Clin Ther. 1999;21(2):281–95.

Duroudier NP, Tulah AS, Sayers I. Leukotriene pathway genetics and pharmacogenetics in allergy. Allergy. 2009;64(6):823–39.

Dykewicz MS, Wallace DV, Amrol DJ, Baroody FM, Bernstein JA, Craig TJ, et al. Rhinitis 2020: a practice parameter update. J Allergy Clin Immunol. 2020;146(4):721–67.

García-García C, Kim M, Baik I. Associations of dietary vitamin A and C intake with asthma, allergic rhinitis, and allergic respiratory diseases. Nutr Res Pract. 2023;17(5):997–1006.

Głowacka K, Wiela-Hojeńska A. Pseudoephedrine – benefits and risks. Int J Mol Sci. 2021;22(10):5146.

Hoyte FCL, Nelson HS. Recent advances in allergic rhinitis. F1000Research. 2018;7:1333.
Johnson DA, Hricik JG. The pharmacology of alpha-adrenergic decongestants. Pharmacotherapy. 1993;13(6 Pt 2):110S–5S.
Kim YH, Kim KW, Kim MJ, Sol IS, Yoon SH, Ahn HS, et al. Vitamin D levels in allergic rhinitis: a systematic review and meta-analysis. Pediatr Allergy Immunol. 2016;27(6):580–90.
Linton S, Hossenbaccus L, Ellis AK. Evidence-based use of antihistamines for treatment of allergic conditions. Ann Allergy Asthma Immunol. 2023;131(4):412–20.
Lopez-Santamarina A, Gonzalez EG, Lamas A, et al. Probiotics as a possible strategy for the prevention and treatment of allergies. Narrat Rev Foods. 2021;10(4):701.
Luo C, Peng S, Li M, Ao X, Liu Z. The efficacy and safety of probiotics for allergic rhinitis: a systematic review and meta-analysis. Front Immunol. 2022:13.
Mitra S, Paul S, Roy S, Sutradhar H, Bin Emran T, Nainu F, et al. Exploring the immune-boosting functions of vitamins and minerals as nutritional food bioactive compounds: a comprehensive review. Molecules. 2022;27(2):555.
Nelson HS. Mechanisms of intranasal steroids in the management of upper respiratory allergic diseases. J Allergy Clin Immunol. 1999;104(4):s138–43.
Özdemir Ö. Various effects of different probiotic strains in allergic disorders: an update from laboratory and clinical data. Clin Exp Immunol. 2010;160(3):295–304.
Simons FER, Simons KJ. Histamine and H1-antihistamines: celebrating a century of progress. J Allergy Clin Immunol. 2011;128(6):1139–50.
Xue CCL, Hugel HM, Li CG, Efficacy SDF. Chemistry and pharmacology of Chinese herbal medicine for allergic rhinitis. Curr Med Chem. 2024;11(11):1403–21.
Yasir M, Goyal A, Sonthalia S. Corticosteroid adverse effects. In: StatPearls. Treasure Island (FL): StatPearls Publishing; 2024. Available from: https://www.ncbi.nlm.nih.gov/books/NBK531462/
Yuko E, Cherian V. Can Eating Local Honey Help With Seasonal Allergies? See What Allergists Say [Internet]. Real Simple. 2024. Available from: https://www.realsimple.com/health/preventative-health/cold-flu-allergies/is-local-honey-good-for-allergies

Chapter 6
Nasal and Ophthalmic Medications for Treatment of Allergic Rhinitis and Allergic Conjunctivitis

Shalakha Bonthu, Nicole Akar-Ghibril, and Christopher Chang

Introduction

Since the primary symptoms of allergic rhinitis (AR), allergic conjunctivitis (AC), or their combination, allergic rhinoconjunctivitis (ARC), involve the nose and/or eyes, it is only fitting that these are the target areas for administration of medications for AR, AC or ARC. For decades, intranasal medications have been the mainstay of AR treatment, ranging from corticosteroids to antihistamines to decongestants. In fact, intranasal corticosteroids are widely considered the first-line treatment for AR. Intraocular medications are also available for the treatment of allergic conjunctivitis specifically. There are also options that are not as well-known such as intranasal cromolyn and intranasal ipratropium. Ophthalmic medicationscan be effective in AC and may in fact help with nasal symptoms as well. This chapter will discuss the mechanism of action, safety, side effects, and recommendations of the mentioned intranasal and ophthalmic medications. The efficacy of monotherapy versus combination therapy of each of these medications will also be explored (Abdullah et al. 2022; Dykewicz et al. 2020; Wallace et al. 2008).

S. Bonthu
Charles E. Schmidt College of Medicine, Florida Atlantic University, Boca Raton, FL, USA

N. Akar-Ghibril · C. Chang (✉)
Division of Immunology, Allergy, and Pediatric Rheumatology, Joe DiMaggio Children's Hospital, Memorial Healthcare System, Hollywood, FL, USA
e-mail: chrchang@mhs.net

M. Mahmoudi (ed.), *Treatment and Management of Allergic Rhinitis*,
https://doi.org/10.1007/978-3-031-88107-7_6

Intranasal Corticosteroids

Intranasal corticosteroids (INCSs) are the first-line monotherapy for persistent moderate to severe AR, especially for those patients whose quality of life is severely impacted. INCSs trigger the synthesis and release of anti-inflammatory proteins while simultaneously inhibiting the synthesis and release of pro-inflammatory molecules. The mechanism of action of corticosteroids involves diffusion of the medication across the cell membrane into the cytoplasm, where it binds to the glucocorticoid receptor. Upon corticosteroid binding, a molecular chaperone protein, such as hsp90, hsp70 and cyclophilin-40 (Cyp-40), which typically prevents transport of the glucocorticoid receptor to the nucleus, dissociates from the newly formed corticosteroid-glucocorticoid receptor complex (Mygind et al. 2001). This complex is then able to cross into the nucleus and bind to DNA sequences called glucocorticoid receptor elementsin the promoters of different genes, thereby increasing transcription of anti-inflammatory molecules. The corticosteroid-glucocorticoid complex can also indirectly reduce gene transcription of pro-inflammatory molecules by interacting with transcription factors that are already present. Overall, this results in greater expression of genes that code for anti-inflammatory molecules while decreasing expression of genes coding for proinflammatory molecules. Since corticosteroids operate at a transcription level rather than directly interacting with already produced proinflammatory molecules or their receptors, the effect is not immediate and can be delayed by hours to days (Fig. 6.1) (Daley-Yates et al. 2021).

A somewhat unknown distinction between first- and second-generation INCSs exists. First-generation INCSs include triamcinolone acetonide, budesonide, flunisolide, dexamethasone, and beclomethasone dipropionate; second-generation INCSs include fluticasone propionate, fluticasone furoate, ciclesonide, and mometasone furoate. While all INCSs are generally considered safe and effective, each one's distinct structure results in different properties (Table 6.1). Different INCSs can have increased or decreased glucocorticoid receptor binding affinity which can affect their therapeutic efficacy as well as their safety profiles. For example, the second-generation INCSs have an increased glucocorticoid receptor selectivity and binding affinity, increased uptake in the nasal tissue, and decreased systemic effects compared to earlier INCSs. A higher glucocorticoid receptor binding affinity is associated with higher nasal tissue uptake and higher topical potency. Consequently, second generation INCSs are associated with lower oral uptake, resulting in lower systemic exposure. Lower systemic exposure is then linked to a higher therapeutic index and fewer adverse effects.A systematic review and network meta-analysis found that among the different intranasal corticosteroids, mometasone furoate has the highest efficacy in treating seasonal AR, followed by fluticasone furoate, ciclesonide, fluticasone propionate, and triamcinolone acetonide. In perennial AR, a network meta-analysis ranked budesonide as having the highest efficacy, followed by fluticasone furoate, triamcinolone acetonide, ciclesonide, and mometasone furoate. Though second-generation INCSs were consistently ranked as some of the most

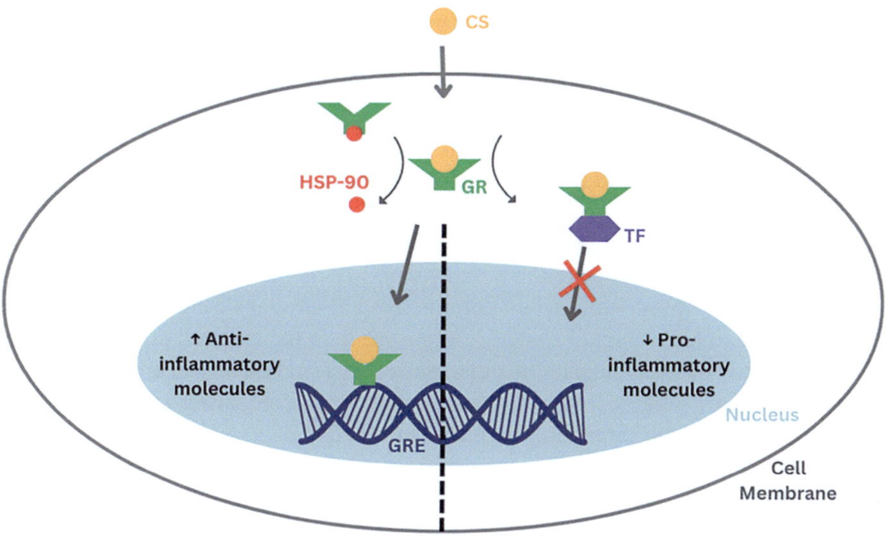

Fig. 6.1 Mechanism of action of corticosteroids (CS). CS diffuses across the cell membrane and binds glucocorticoid receptor (GR). Heat shock protein (HSP-90) dissociates from the glucocorticoid receptor. The CS-GR complex diffuses across the nuclear membrane and binds to glucocorticoid receptor elements (GRE), increasing transcription of anti-inflammatory molecules. Another pathway involves the CS-GR complex instead binding a transcription factor (TF), such as NF-kB, to reduce the transcription of pro-inflammatory molecules

Table 6.1 Relative properties of first-generation v. second-generation intranasal corticosteroids

Properties	First-generation INCSs	Second-generation INCSs
Glucocorticoid receptor selectivity and binding affinity	Lower	Higher
Uptake in nasal tissue	Lower	Higher
Topical potency	Lower	Higher
Oral uptake	Higher	Lower
Systemic exposure	Higher	Lower

efficacious medications for different types of AR, they are not always superior to first-generation INCSs.

All FDA-approved INCSs are currently delivered in the form of metered-dose nasal spray pumps, pressurized metered-dose inhalers, nasal drops, and exhalation delivery system (EDS). None are currently administered in the form of nasal irrigation, dry powder devices, or nebulizing solution. One INCS, fluticasone propionate, is available as a metered-dose spray pump and as an EDS device, the most popular brands being Flonase® and Xhance®, respectively. Flonase® can be found over the counter and treats allergies, while Xhance® is a prescription-only medication that is FDA-approved for the treatment of chronic rhinosinusitis with and without nasal polyps (Messina et al. 2019). Flonase® is also available in generic form. Metered-dose spray pumps have been popular for decades due to their ease of use. EDS devices, on the other hand, use a newer delivery method that is designed with the intent to have the drug reach deeper into the nose, thereby leading to higher efficacy of the drug.

EDS devices are activated when the patient blows through the mouthpiece, which is connected to the intranasal medication reservoir and allows the drug to enter the nostril. A randomized comparison of fluticasone propionate metered dose spray pump and fluticasone propionate EDS device concluded that the EDS device produced a significantly higher relative bioavailability of fluticasone propionate than the metered dose spray pump when administered at similar dosages. However, the EDS device also led to higher systemic exposure than the metered dose spray, so it is important to consider the patient's disease severity and quality of life in deciding which to use. The same recommendation applies when comparing any dosages and delivery devices of the same drug (Rollema et al. 2022).

INCSs are considered safe because they do not have significant systemic absorption and, as such, generally do not cause any systemic adverse effects. Local side effects include dryness, burning, epistaxis, and rarely, septal perforations. There have been reports of an impact on short-term growth in children using INCSs, but no effects on long-term growth nor the hypothalamic-pituitary-adrenal axis have been found in more recent studies (Mener et al. 2015). It is not just the delivered dose of INCSs that determines the effects of systemic exposure. Pharmacokinetic and pharmacodynamic differences between different INCSs and among patients need to be factored in to reach real-world conclusions on efficacy and safety. Nevertheless, the lowest effective dose should always be prescribed to patients with AR. Most INCSs can be used safely in pregnancy, but in one Canadian prospective cohort study, triamcinolone was associated with congenital respiratory defects, so caution should be exercised when prescribing to pregnant patients.

One additional factor to consider is the hazards of unintentional exposure of topical steroids in the eye. Use of potent topical corticosteroids in the periorbital region have been shown to lead to glaucoma and cataracts (Daniel & Orchard 2015). However, for application on areas of the face besides the periorbital region, there is no substantial evidence that it can lead to glaucoma and cataracts. There have been some case reports of older patients developing posterior subcapsular cataracts after INCS use. However, a meta-analysis of 10 different clinical trials (total of 2226 patients studied) did not confirm any association between the two. The meta-analysis also did not show any increased risk of higher intraocular pressure after INCS use (Valenzuela et al. 2019). Regardless, it is best practice to keep watch for the development of these issues when using any steroids on the face (Soe et al. 2023).

Overall, INCSs are often the first-choice medication for treating AR, due to their favorable safety profile and demonstrated efficacy. INCSs can take anywhere from several hours to multiple days to take full effect, so it is important to emphasize the importance of therapy adherence to patients to achieve optimal results.

Intranasal and Ocular Antihistamines

Intranasal antihistamines (INAHs) and oral antihistamines target the H1 receptor. However, INAHs have been found to have equal or superior efficacy compared to oral antihistamines, and they are recommended if oral antihistamines cannot sufficiently treat symptoms. This is likely because intranasal administration has been found to result in higher nasal tissue levels of the compound. INAHs also have a more rapid onset of action (15–30 min) than INCSs and oral antihistamines, and they are more effective in treating nasal congestion compared to oral antihistamines (Berger et al. 2016). Compared to INCSs, INAHs are equally or slightly inferior in treating nasal symptoms, but they have comparable efficacy in treating ocular symptoms. INAHs are considered first-line treatment for seasonal AR and intermittent AR. INAHs are also regarded as first-line treatment for mild AR, while INCSs are first-line treatment for moderate to severe AR (Yanez & Rodrigo 2002).

Two of the most used antihistamines for treatment of AR are azelastine and olopatadine. Both have been FDA-approved for seasonal AR with similar efficacy, while azelastine is also FDA-approved for perennial AR. Azelastine not only binds to H1 receptors with high affinity, but also inhibits H2 receptors and expression of inflammatory mediators, and it desensitizes transient receptor potential vanilloid 1 (TRPV1) ion channels. Azelastine is commonly associated with a bitter taste that lasts up to 30 min after administration. Fortunately, this can be averted with different formulations of the compound, such as by adding sucralose. Intranasal and ocular olopatadine, on the other hand, also have inhibitory effects on mast cell degranulation. Intranasal olopatadine can cause a bitter taste and epistaxis, but it is less frequently associated with somnolence than azelastine.

Levocabastine and ketotifen are two other antihistamines that have been explored thoroughly as viable treatments for AR (Okubo et al. 2010). Levocabastine nasal spray is proven to be safe and effective for both perennial AR and seasonal AR (Hampel et al. 1999). Ocular ketotifen is preferred over its oral form as it is just as effective but creates fewer systemic complications compared to oral ketotifen. Both levocabastine and ketotifen are also mast cell stabilizers (Akhavan et al. 2015).

INAH should be used with caution in pregnant individuals, as trials regarding safety in pregnancy have not yet been conducted and data is scarce. In all cases, benefit to risk analysis should be performed prior to the use of any medication.

Intranasal Decongestants

Nasal decongestants are alpha-adrenergic agonists that cause vasoconstriction in the nasal mucosa to decrease inflammation. Commonly used nasal decongestants include oxymetazoline, phenylephrine, and xylometazoline. These agents can provide up to 10 h of relief from nasal congestion by improving nasal resistance, increasing nasal cross-sectional areas, and increasing nasal airflow. However, they do not affect symptoms such as itching, nasal secretion, and sneezing, and they do not directly inhibit the release of inflammatory mediators due to allergen exposure. In the short term and in certain situations, an intranasal decongestant may be helpful if administered with an INCS. This is particularly true in patients with such severe mucosal edema that other intranasal agents cannot be delivered.

Side effects of nasal decongestants can include local burning, sneezing, and dryness.Serious adverse effects of nasal decongestants include the development of alpha-receptor tachyphylaxis and rhinitis medicamentosa (Mortuaire et al. 2013). Tachyphylaxis is the phenomenon in whichthere is a sudden, acute decrease in the responsiveness to a drug, oftentimes after prolonged drug use. This often leads to excessive use of nasal decongestants which then results in rebound congestion, a condition known as rhinitis medicamentosa. Studies on rhinitis medicamentosa have been primarily conducted in animals or healthy individuals, and results have been variable with some subjects developing rhinitis medicamentosa after only 3 days and others not even after 6 weeks of use. However, in view of the risk of rebound congestion, nasal decongestants are only recommended for short-term use and under the guidance of a physician.

Nasal decongestants are also contraindicated in patients of any age with hypertension, thyroid disease, and heart disease. They are generally not recommended forchildren.As for pregnant individuals, decongestants can present with some risks. The Sloan Birth Defects Study found that topical decongestants were associated with gastroschisis and pyloric stenosis when used during the first trimester. When used during the second trimester, there was an association with renal collecting system anomalies. It is true that oral decongestants have been found to have much higher rate of serious adverse effects compared to intranasal decongestants, likely because oral medications typically have greater systemic effects than intranasal medications. However, since the relative benefit of congestion relief does not outweigh the risk of such teratogenic effects, it is recommended that intranasal decongestants are avoided as best as possible during pregnancy, especially during the first trimester.

In conclusion, nasal decongestants are helpful in relieving nasal congestion. However, due to the risk of rhinitis medicamentosa and its severe potential effects during pregnancy, regular or maintenance usage should be avoided. Nasal decongestants should be treated only as a short-term solution for nasal congestion, and alternative long-term treatment options should be sought out when feasible.

Nasal Saline

Nasal saline irrigation uses saline solutions to moisturize nasal passages, remove allergens and irritants like dust and pollen, and eliminate mucus. It can be administered via sprays, irrigation pots, bottles, and pumps. Optimal volume, temperature, frequency of administration, alkalinity, and tonicity of the solution have not yet been determined. Side effects such as irritation are minimal, and epistaxis has not been reported as an adverse effect in several trials (Wang et al. 2020).

With tap water use, there is a risk of transmission of the amoeba *Naegleria fowleri*, which can cause fatal primary amebic meningoencephalitis. To prevent this, the U.S. FDA Centers for Disease Control and Prevention recommends boiling tap water for 1–5 min and then cooling before use in nasal irrigation. Alternatively, patients can buy distilled or sterile water, use bottled water, or boil or pass tap water through a filter (CDC 2024).

Nasal saline irrigation has been shown to be a safe adjunctive treatment along with medication in treating AR in adults and children, as there is evidence that patient-reported symptom severity is lower when using saline irrigation than not. However, it has not been proven to be more effective than use of pharmacologic intervention alone in adults. In children, it can be used as an adjunctivetherapy to medication in treating AR, and it can be a first-line treatment during pregnancy. Overall, saline irrigation is a cheap, accessible, and safe option for treatment of AR, but it may not be as effective as other monotherapies.

Intranasal Capsaicin

Capsaicin (8-methyl-N-vanillyl-6-nonenamide), a compound in chili peppers that contributes to their spicy nature, has long been used in the treatment of obesity, cancer, dermatologic conditions, cardiovascular conditions, and gastrointestinal conditions. Though not approved by the FDA, capsaicin has also been used for treatment of idiopathic rhinitis, as topical application to nasal mucosa has been shown to reduce nasal congestion, sinus pain, postnasal discharge, and rhinorrhea (Toukan et al. 2022). Capsaicin is a selective TRPV1 ion channel agonist that stimulates afferent nerves of nociceptive C fibers and A-delta fibers. After this initial stimulation, these neurons become unresponsive to stimuli due to a long refractory period, explaining capsaicin's mechanism of action and therapeutic potential (Cheng et al. 2006; Fokkens et al. 2016).

Currently, there is no consensus as to whether capsaicin is an effective treatment for AR. Some studies have shown a reduction in AR symptoms while others have not shown any significant therapeutic benefits. In terms of safety and adverse reactions, side effects of topical capsaicin can include burning, irritation, erythema, and pain at the site of application. Capsaicin has not been found to be harmful for pregnant individuals; in fact, a small study found that topical capsaicin can be used safely as treatment for nausea and vomiting during pregnancy (Murphy et al. 2023). Overall, capsaicin's efficacy in treating AR can only be determined with future well-constructed randomized controlled trials, assessing the impact of different dosages, locations of treatment, and modes of administration.

Intranasal Ipratropium Bromide

During activation of the parasympathetic nervous system, acetylcholine is released and binds muscarinic receptors on nasal glands, resulting in increased nasal secretions. Patients with perennial AR have cholinergic hyperactivity. Ipratropium bromide is an anticholinergic compound that selectively binds to these muscarinic receptors, allowing for the reduction of nasal symptoms due to anti-secretory properties when administered intranasally at the nasal mucosa. Intranasal ipratropium bromide has specifically been found to be effective for anterior rhinorrhea. Side effects of intranasal ipratropium bromide can include epistaxis and nasal dryness, as with many other intranasal agents, but it is well-tolerated overall and has not shown any clinically significant systemic effects. This is also the reason why acute overdose is unlikely. Oral ipratropium bromide, on the other hand, has more systemic effects. The safety of intranasal ipratropium bromide use in pregnancy has yet to be determined. Preliminary animal studies have been conducted, but due to limited evidence, ipratropium bromide should only be used during pregnancy when very clearly indicated. With a rapid onset of action of just 15 min, intranasal ipratropium is an effective choice of treatment for patients with perennial AR who have rhinorrhea as one of their primary symptoms (Kaiser et al. 1995).

Intranasal and Ocular Cromolyn Sodium

Cromolyn sodium is derived from a furanochromone called khellin, which comes from the herb *Ammi visnaga*. Administered intranasally, ocularly, and orally, cromolyn sodium reduces the release of inflammatory mediators by inhibiting the degranulation of sensitized mast cells, thus reducing symptoms of AR (Meltzer 2002). Cromolyn has minimal side effects and is considered safe in pregnancy as it is poorly absorbed systematically and has not been associated with any drug interactions. This likely explains its availability as an over-the-counter medication. Intranasal cromolyn sodium is approved for adults and children ages 2 years and older. Cromolyn sodium has been shown to prevent symptoms on a short-term basis, particularly when used prophylactically (Spector 1989). Though intranasal cromolyn sodium has proven to be efficacious in treating symptoms of AR (specifically seasonal AR and perennial AR), studies show it has similar efficacy when compared to oral antihistamines and is not as effective as intranasal corticosteroids. Patients may have to concurrently use a nasal decongestant with intranasal cromolyn sodium if they have significant nasalo bstruction. Therefore, intranasal cromolyn sodium should be recommended primarily as an option for use just before episodic allergen exposure. Ocular cromolyn sodium is recommended for those who have allergic eye symptoms, specifically when conjunctivitis is present (Orgel et al. 1991; Welsh et al. 1987).

INCS and INAH Combination Therapy

While INCSs are the first-line monotherapy in treating AR, it is also worthwhile exploring the efficacy of combination therapy. INCSs combined with INAHs are a well-researched pairing since both are considered some of the best treatments for AR (Carr et al. 2012). Multiple different double-blind placebo-controlled studies, with patients of ages 12 or older, tested combination therapy with INCSs paired with INAHs. Studies have determined that the combination of an INCS with an INAH should be used to treat patients ages 12 or older in two different scenarios: if a patient with seasonal AR has moderate to severe nasal symptoms, and if a patient with seasonal AR or perennial AR has symptoms that have been resistant to monotherapy. These studies showed that the combination of an INCS with an INAH has a faster onset than either individual therapy, and that dual therapy is also more effective in reducing total symptoms than either agent alone. These results were also supported in one trial with children ages 6–11 years. It is important to note that these studies examined combination therapy as an initial treatment rather than as an add-on. However, data from other studies supports the recommendation that combination therapy of both an INCS and INAH should be used if a patient is resistant to monotherapy with only one of these medications (Gross et al. 2019).

The combination of INCSs and INAHs has not always been found to be superior to INCS monotherapy. This is because INCSs and INAHs have some opposing pharmacological properties. For example, INAHs are in a hydrophilic solution while INCSs are in a lipophilic solution. If an INCS is applied first, it leaves a lipid layer on the nasal mucous membranes. Any INAH that is applied afterwards would then not be able to penetrate this layer, resulting in minimal effect from the INAH. However, two fixed combinations of INCS and INAHs have emerged over the years that do provide a therapeutic benefit compared to INCS monotherapy.

Fixed combinations have the advantage of combining the rapid onset of action of INAHs with the superior efficacy of INCSs, unlike free combinations that can have mixed results or few additional benefits. The first fixed combination of INCS and INAH that has been proven to have a superior effect compared to monotherapy is MP29-02, trade name Dymista® (Meltzer et al. 2012; Meltzer et al. 2013), which contains fluticasone propionate (INCS) and azelastine (INAH) (Hampel et al. 2010; Meltzer et al. 2012). An RCT that studied patients with moderate to severe seasonal AR found that patients experienced an onset of relief of approximately 30 min, and they experienced significantly more nasal symptom relief, especially nasal congestion, when treated with Dymista® compared to INCS or INAH monotherapy. Headache (3.1%), dysgeusia (2.1%), epistaxis (1.5%), and mucosal erosion (1.5%) were some adverse side effects that were reported in the Dymista® group, but this reflected a similar safety profile to those of azelastine and fluticasone. In fact, dysgeusia was reported in 2.1% of patients in the Dymista® group and in 7.2% of the azelastine group, which is important to consider with patient adherence to treatment. Dymista® is currently FDA-approved for children ages 6 years and older.

Another fixed combination of INCS and INAH that has been FDA-approved for patients ages 12 years and older is Ryaltris®, the generic being a combination of olopatadinehydrochloride and mometasone furoate. Trials testing for dosage found that two sprays per nostril of the generic compound twice a day showed significant clinical improvement compared to either olopatadine or mometasone alone.One phase III clinical trial of olopatadine-mometasone conducted by Gross et al. tested 1176 participants ages 12 and older in a double-blind, placebo-controlled study. The results concluded that olopatadine-mometasone is efficacious for treating nasal and ocular symptoms of seasonal AR and has an onset of action of 15 min. A different study by Segall et al. held over 52 weeks found that olopatadine-mometasone was well-tolerated and resulted in significant symptom relief with an onset of action of 15 min. Adverse reactions included dysgeusia. Olopatadine-mometasone has not been studied in pregnancy or in breastfeeding, so use in these patients should involve careful benefit-risk considerations (Hampel et al.2019).

When comparing the two FDA-approved INCS and INAH fixed combination therapies, Dymista® and Ryaltris®, there are a few differences. Compared to Dymista®, symptom relief from Ryaltris®treatment was not significantly different, but both demonstrated statistically significant improvement of symptoms compared to a placebo. However, studies have shown that participants preferred the olopatadine-mometasone combination over fluticasone-azelastine when it came to sensory properties of the products. To increase adherence, patients who value sensory properties when choosing their treatment should consider using Ryaltris®. On the other hand, Dymista® is preferable for those who would like a less rigid treatment regimen with just one spray per nostril twice a day instead of two sprays per nostril twice daily. Other different combinations of INCSs and INAHs that have not been FDA-approved yet are undergoing clinical trials.

Additional Combination Therapies

INCSs combined with INAHs is the most well-known form of combination therapy for AR treatment. However, there are other combination therapies available, including INCSs with intranasal decongestants, INCSs with intranasal ipratropium bromide, INCSs with oral antihistamines, and INCSs with oral leukotriene receptor antagonists.

Depending on specific persistent nasal symptoms, certain combination therapies may be a better option compared to monotherapy. For example, administering an intranasal decongestant for a patient already taking an INCS can be beneficial if they have persistent nasal congestion. However, as mentioned when discussing intranasal decongestants, these should only be used as a short-term treatment to prevent development of rhinitis medicamentosa. On the other hand, if a patient taking an INCS has persistent rhinorrhea rather than persistent nasal congestion, then administering intranasal ipratropium bromide concurrently can improve the patient's rhinorrhea. Though no drug interactions have been observed in these two combinations, it is still important to closely monitor patients using any combination therapy to ensure both safety and efficacy.

Despite these circumstances in which combining INCSs with another therapy can be beneficial, such is not always the case. Combining INCSs with oral antihistamines is not preferred over INCS monotherapy. A review showed that there was no significantly increased symptom relief with the combination of INCSs and oral antihistamines compared to INCS monotherapy. Similarly, combining INCSs with oral leukotriene receptor antagonists lacks well-controlled trials, and this combination also presents the threat of neuropsychiatric complications that can accompany the use of montelukast. Therefore, in this case, it would be safer to administer the INCS alone. As for intranasal decongestants paired with intranasal ipratropium bromide, there is no robust published literature on the effects of this combination.

When discussing combination therapies, there is a clear preference for using INCSs with INAHs to treat moderate to severe AR that is resistant to monotherapy. Combining INCSs with intranasal ipratropium bromide or with intranasal decongestants can help combat rhinorrhea and nasal congestion, respectively. Any other combination has insufficient evidence to prove its superiority over monotherapy or it has already been proven to not have any statistical difference in symptom management. Regardless, monotherapy should still be the initial treatment option, and combination therapies should be considered on a case-by-case basis, accounting for disease severity, patient preference, cost, and patient adherence.

Additional Factors to Consider When Choosing Appropriate Therapy

The main deciding factor for choosing a specific treatment is its efficacy, but that cannot be the only attribute that is assessed. Beyond the effectiveness of each type of intranasal and ophthalmic medication, it is important to consider each patient's preference, financial circumstances, and lifestyle choices when selecting the appropriate treatment. If a patient has hypergeusia, a foul taste may deter them from adhering well to treatment, even in the face of ongoing symptoms. Patients with very busy schedules may have a difficult time committing to a treatment that requires multiple administrations daily. Even a cost difference of a few dollars can add up over the months and take a toll on some patients. As physicians, it is crucial to identify the patient's priorities and treat them accordingly.

The debate of whether to use monotherapy or combination therapy has many layers to it. Starting with monotherapy is not only more cost-effective than combination therapy, but it is also more convenient since patients are only responsible for one medication, which increases patient adherence. Combination therapy also presents a higher risk for adverse effects. Within options for combination therapy, a singular dual-medication device is typically more expensive compared to the cost of two individual medications. Combination therapy in a single device is not always covered by many insurance carriers.

The potential lower cost of separating combination therapy into two or more devices is accompanied by the inconvenience of having to use two separate medications. These must be administered a few minutes apart to allow for adequate absorption of each medication, so there is a chance that patient adherence may decrease. Aside from costs, patient preferences also play a role in the decision. For example, some patients may ask to start with two medications instead of monotherapy in hopes that combination therapy will cause greater symptom relief, despite a lack of evidence supporting this treatment regimen.

When choosing between oral route and nasal sprays, patients may personally prefer one or the other regardless of relative efficacy. Some will prefer topical agents over oral agents, and others find nasal sprays create an uncomfortable sensation. Depending on their lifestyle, they may prefer a medication with a shorter or longer onset of action, or they prefer to use one long-lasting medication instead of frequently administering throughout the day. Using medications that are over-the-counter and therefore more easily accessible may also be a priority for the patient who values cost effectiveness and limiting trips to their physician's office.

When making the final decision about treatment options, it is crucial that patient lifestyle, adherence, and all the factors discussed above are considered to not only reduce disease severity but to also prioritize quality of life and patient adherence. Table 6.2 shows recommended dosages of the medications in the different classes discussed above.

Summary and Conclusion

In summary, the list of nasal and ophthalmic medications for the treatment of AR is extensive, each with its own strengths and drawbacks. Intranasal corticosteroids remain the first choice of treatment for AR, but intranasal antihistamines are now the preferred treatment for seasonal AR and intermittent AR. Nasal saline irrigation presents a safe, effective option for patients of all demographics, including those who are pregnant. Intranasal ipratropium bromide is conditionally recommended due to its risk for complications when used long-term, and intranasal and ocular cromolyn sodium are conditionally recommended only for episodic allergen exposure. Intranasal capsaicin, while generally safe and effective, needs more evidence to support its promotion to being an approved treatment for AR. As for combination therapy, INCSs can be used concurrently with INAHs for patients who have been unresponsive to monotherapy. INCSs can also be used with an intranasal decongestant or intranasal ipratropium bromide to combat persistent nasal congestion and rhinorrhea, respectively, but with nasal decongestants, the possibility of rhinitis medicamentosa should always be considered.

Though there is already a great deal of research regarding nasal and ophthalmic medications for AR, future research should aim to explore more combination therapies. Which specific INCS combined with which specific INAH would be the most effective in treating unresponsive patients? Would nasal saline irrigation with an

Table 6.2 Dosages of nasal and ophthalmic medications for allergic rhinitis

Drug class	Generic drug	Dosage
First-generation intranasal corticosteroids	Budesonide	12 years and older: 2 sprays (32 mcg per spray) per nostril once daily, reduce to 1 spray per nostril once daily after symptom improvement 6–11 years: 1 spray (32 mcg per spray) per nostril once daily, can increase to 2 sprays per nostril once daily if no symptom improvement and then reduce back to 1 spray per nostril once daily after symptom improvement
	Flunisolide	15 years and older: 2 sprays (25 mcg per spray) per nostril twice daily, or three times daily if needed 6–14 years: 1 spray (25 mcg per spray) per nostril three times daily or 2 sprays per nostril twice daily
	Triamcinolone acetonide	12 years and older: 2 sprays (55 mcg per spray) per nostril once daily 6–11 years: 1 spray (55 mcg per spray) per nostril once daily, can increase to 2 sprays per nostril once daily if no symptom improvement 2- < 6 years of age: 1 spray (55 mcg per spray) per nostril once daily
Second-generation intranasal corticosteroids	Fluticasone furoate	12 years and older: Up to 2 sprays (27.5 mcg per spray) per nostril once daily 2–11 years: 1 spray (27.5 mcg per spray) per nostril once daily
	Fluticasone propionate	12 years and older: Up to 2 sprays (50 mcg per spray) per nostril once daily 4–11 years: 1 spray (50 mcg per spray) per nostril once daily
	Mometasone furoate	12 years and older: 2 sprays (50 mcg per spray) per nostril once daily 2–11 years: 1 spray (50 mcg per spray) per nostril once daily
Intranasal antihistamines	Azelastine hydrochloride	12 years and older: Up to 2 sprays (137–205.5 mcg per spray) per nostril twice daily 6–11 years: 1 spray (137 mcg per spray) per nostril twice daily >6 months - < 6 years: 1 spray (137mcg/spray) per nostril twice daily (limited data available)
	Olopatadine hydrochloride	12 years and older: 2 sprays (665 mcg per spray) per nostril twice daily 6–11 years: 1 spray (665 mcg per spray) per nostril twice daily

(continued)

Table 6.2 (continued)

Drug class	Generic drug	Dosage
Ocular antihistamines	Ketotifen	3 years and older: 1 eye drop (0.025% ketotifen) in each affected eye twice daily, 8–12 hours apart, no more than twice per day
	Olopatadine hydrochloride	2 years and older: 1 eye drop (0.1% olopatadine) in each affected eye twice daily, 6–8 hours apart, no more than twice per day OR 1 eye drop (0.2% olopatadine) in each affected eye once daily, no more than once per day OR 1 drop (0.7% olopatadine) in each affected eye once daily
Intranasal decongestants	Oxymetazoline hydrochloride	6 years and older: 2 or 3 sprays (0.05% oxymetazoline hydrochloride) per nostril, not more often than every 10–12 h, no more than twice in any 24 h period, for up to 3 days duration
	Phenylephrine hydrochloride	6 years and older: 2 or 3 sprays (0.25–1% phenylephrine hydrochloride) per nostril, not more often than every 4 h, for up to 3 days duration 2- < 6 years: 0.125% solution: 1 drop in each nostril every 2–4 h as needed
	Xylometazoline hydrochloride	Adults: 2 sprays (0.1% xylometazoline hydrochloride) per nostril, not more often than every 8–10 h, for up to 3 days duration
Anticholinergics	Ipratropium bromide	6 years and older: 2 sprays (21 mcg per spray) per nostril two to three times daily OR 5 years and older: 2 sprays (84 mcg per spray) per nostril four times daily, for up to 3 weeks duration
Cromolyn sodium	Intranasal cromolyn sodium	2 years and older: 1 spray (5.2 mg per spray) per nostril, every 4–6 h, three to four times daily, no more than 6 times a day
	Ocular cromolyn sodium	4 years and older: 1 or 2 eye drops (4% cromolyn sodium/1.6 mg cromolyn sodium per drop) in each affected eye 4–6 times daily at regular intervals
INCS-INAH combination	Fluticasone propionate and azelastine hydrochloride (Dymista®)	6 years and older: 1 spray (137 mcg of azelastine hydrochloride and 50 mcg of fluticasone propionate per spray) per nostril twice daily
	Olopatadine hydrochloride and mometasone furoate (Ryaltris®)	12 years and older: 2 sprays (665 mcg of olopatadine hydrochloride and 25 mcg of mometasone furoate per spray) per nostril twice daily 6- < 12 years: 1 spray per nostril twice daily

ophthalmic medication be sufficient in reducing both nasal and ocular symptoms? How effective would it be to combine INAHs with any other class of medications besides INCSs? In the era of personalized medicine, identifying the clinical phenotype most responsive to a respective therapy would be an important area of research for the future.

References

Abdullah B, Latiff AHA, Manuel AM, Jamli FM, Singh HSD, Ismail IH, Jahendran J, Saniasiaya J, Woo KCK, Khoo PC, Singh K, Mohammad N, Mohamad S, Husain S, Mösges R. Pharmacological management of allergic rhinitis: a consensus statement from the Malaysian society of allergy and immunology. J Asthma Allergy. 2022;15:983–1003. https://doi.org/10.2147/JAA.S374346.

Akhavan A, Karimi-Sari H, Khosravi MH, Arefzadeh E, Yavarahmadi M. Comparing the effects of ketotifen fumarate eye drops and ketotifen oral pills on symptom severity and quality of life in patients with allergic rhinitis: a double-blind randomized clinical trial. Int Forum Allergy Rhinol. 2015;5(5):386–91. https://doi.org/10.1002/alr.21491.

Berger W, Bousquet J, Fox AT, Just J, Muraro A, Nieto A, Valovirta E, Wickman M, Wahn U. MP-AzeFlu is more effective than fluticasone propionate for the treatment of allergic rhinitis in children. Allergy. 2016;71(8):1219–22. https://doi.org/10.1111/all.12903.

Carr W, Bernstein J, Lieberman P, Meltzer E, Bachert C, Price D, Munzel U, Bousquet J. A novel intranasal therapy of azelastine with fluticasone for the treatment of allergic rhinitis. J Allergy Clin Immunol. 2012;129(5):1282–1289.e10. https://doi.org/10.1016/j.jaci.2012.01.077.

CDC. How to prevent Naegleria fowleri infection when rinsing sinuses or nasal passages. Centers for Disease Control and Prevention; 2024, May 14. https://www.cdc.gov/naegleria/prevention/sinus-rinsing.html

Cheng J, Yang XN, Liu X, Zhang SP. Capsaicin for allergic rhinitis in adults. Cochrane Database Syst Rev. 2006;2006(2):CD004460. https://doi.org/10.1002/14651858.CD004460.pub2.

Daley-Yates PT, Larenas-Linnemann D, Bhargave C, Verma M. Intranasal corticosteroids: topical potency, systemic activity and therapeutic index. J Asthma Allergy. 2021;14:1093–104. https://doi.org/10.2147/JAA.S321332.

Daniel BS, Orchard D. Ocular side–effects of topical corticosteroids: what a dermatologist needs to know. Australas J Dermatol. 2015;56(3):164–9. https://doi.org/10.1111/ajd.12292.

Dykewicz MS, Wallace DV, Amrol DJ, Baroody FM, Bernstein JA, Craig TJ, Dinakar C, Ellis AK, Finegold I, Golden DBK, Greenhawt MJ, Hagan JB, Horner CC, Khan DA, Lang DM, Larenas-Linnemann DES, Lieberman JA, Meltzer EO, Oppenheimer JJ, et al. Rhinitis 2020: a practice parameter update. J Allergy Clin Immunol. 2020;146(4):721–67. https://doi.org/10.1016/j.jaci.2020.07.007.

Fokkens W, Hellings P, Segboer C. Capsaicin for rhinitis. Curr Allergy Asthma Rep. 2016;16:60. https://doi.org/10.1007/s11882-016-0638-1.

Gross GN, Berman G, Amar NJ, Caracta CF, Tantry SK. Efficacy and safety of olopatadine-mometasone combination nasal spray for the treatment of seasonal allergic rhinitis. Ann Allergy Asthma Immunol. 2019;122(6):630–8. https://doi.org/10.1016/j.anai.2019.03.017.

Hampel FC, Martin BG, Dolen J, Travers S, Karcher K, Holton D. Efficacy and safety of levocabastine nasal spray for seasonal allergic rhinitis. Am J Rhinol. 1999;13(1):55–62. https://doi.org/10.2500/105065899781389867.

Hampel FC, Ratner PH, Van Bavel J, Amar NJ, Daftary P, Wheeler W, Sacks H. Double-blind, placebo-controlled study of azelastine and fluticasone in a single nasal spray delivery device. Ann Allergy Asthma Immunol. 2010;105(2):168–73. https://doi.org/10.1016/j.anai.2010.06.008.

Hampel FC, Pedinoff AJ, Jacobs RL, Caracta CF, Tantry SK. Olopatadine-mometasone combination nasal spray: evaluation of efficacy and safety in patients with seasonal allergic rhinitis. Allergy Asthma Proc. 2019;40(4):261–72. https://doi.org/10.2500/aap.2019.40.4223.

Kaiser HB, Findlay SR, Georgitis JW, Grossman J, Ratner PH, Tinkelman DG, Roszko P, Zegarelli E, Wood CC. Long-term treatment of perennial allergic rhinitis with ipratropium bromide nasal spray 0.06%. J Allergy Clin Immunol. 1995;95(5):1128–32. https://doi.org/10.1016/S0091-6749(95)70217-2.

Meltzer EO. Efficacy and patient satisfaction with cromolyn sodium nasal solution in the treatment of seasonal allergic rhinitis: a placebo-controlled study. Clin Ther. 2002;24(6):942–52. https://doi.org/10.1016/S0149-2918(02)80009-1.

Meltzer EO, LaForce C, Ratner P, Price D, Ginsberg D, Carr W. MP29-02 (a novel intranasal formulation of azelastine hydrochloride and fluticasone propionate) in the treatment of seasonal allergic rhinitis: a randomized, double-blind, placebo-controlled trial of efficacy and safety. Allergy Asthma Proc. 2012;33(4):324–32. https://doi.org/10.2500/aap.2012.33.3587.

Meltzer EO, Ratner P, Bachert C, Carr W, Berger W, Canonica GW, Hadley J, Lieberman P, Hampel FC, Mullol J, Munzel U, Price D, Scadding G, Virchow JC, Wahn U, Murray R, Bousquet J. Clinically relevant effect of a new intranasal therapy (MP29-02) in allergic rhinitis assessed by responder analysis. Int Arch Allergy Immunol. 2013;161(4):369–77. https://doi.org/10.1159/000351404.

Mener DJ, Shargorodsky J, Varadhan R, Lin SY. Topical intranasal corticosteroids and growth velocity in children: a meta-analysis. Int Forum Allergy Rhinol. 2015;5(2):95–103. https://doi.org/10.1002/alr.21430.

Messina JC, Offman E, Carothers JL, Mahmoud RA. A randomized comparison of the pharmacokinetics and bioavailability of fluticasone propionate delivered via Xhance exhalation delivery system versus Flonase nasal spray and Flovent HFA inhalational aerosol. Clin Ther. 2019;41(11):2343–56. https://doi.org/10.1016/j.clinthera.2019.09.013.

Mortuaire G, de Gabory L, François M, Massé G, Bloch F, Brion N, Jankowski R, Serrano E. Rebound congestion and rhinitis medicamentosa: nasal decongestants in clinical practice. Critical review of the literature by a medical panel. Eur Ann Otorhinolaryngol Head Neck Dis. 2013;130(3):137–44. https://doi.org/10.1016/j.anorl.2012.09.005.

Murphy LM, Whelan AR, Griffin LB, Hamel MS. A pilot randomized control trial of topical capsaicin as adjunctive therapy for nausea and vomiting of pregnancy. Am J Obst Gynecol MFM. 2023;5(7):100997. https://doi.org/10.1016/j.ajogmf.2023.100997.

Mygind N, Nielsen LP, Hoffmann H-J, Shukla A, Blumberga G, Dahl R, Jacobi H. Mode of action of intranasal corticosteroids. J Allergy Clin Immunol. 2001;108(1):S16–25. https://doi.org/10.1067/mai.2001.115561.

Okubo K, Uchida E, Nogami S. Levocabastine nasal spray significantly improves perennial allergic rhinitis: a single-blind placebo-controlled study. Auris Nasus Larynx. 2010;37(4):436–42. https://doi.org/10.1016/j.anl.2009.11.014.

Orgel HA, Meltzer EO, Kemp JP, Ostrom NK, Welch MJ. Comparison of intranasal cromolyn sodium, 4%, and oral terfenadine for allergic rhinitis: symptoms, nasal cytology, nasal ciliary clearance, and rhinomanometry. Ann Allergy Asthma Immunol. 1991;66(3):234–44.

Rollema C, van Roon EN, van Boven JFM, Hagedoorn P, Klemmeier T, Kocks JH, Metting EI, Oude Elberink HNG, Peters TTA, San Giorgi MRM, de Vries TW. Pharmacology, particle deposition and drug administration techniques of intranasal corticosteroids for treating allergic rhinitis. Clin Exp Allergy. 2022;52(11):1247–63. https://doi.org/10.1111/cea.14212.

Soe KK, Krikeerati T, Pheerapanyawaranun C, Niyomnaitham S, Phinyo P, Thongngarm T. Comparative efficacy and acceptability of licensed dose intranasal corticosteroids for moderate-to-severe allergic rhinitis: a systematic review and network meta-analysis. Front Pharmacol. 2023;14:1184552. https://doi.org/10.3389/fphar.2023.1184552.

Spector SL. Ocular, nasal and oral cromolyn sodium in the management of non-asthmatic allergic problems. Allergy Proc. 1989;10(3):191–5. https://doi.org/10.2500/108854189778960135.

Toukan N, Kulnik ST, Lewko A, ElShaer A. Therapeutic applications of capsaicin in humans to target conditions of the respiratory system: a scoping review. Respir Med. 2022;194:106772. https://doi.org/10.1016/j.rmed.2022.106772.

Valenzuela CV, Liu JC, Vila PM, Simon L, Doering M, Lieu JEC. Intranasal corticosteroids do not Lead to ocular changes: a systematic review and meta-analysis. Laryngoscope. 2019;129(1):6–12. https://doi.org/10.1002/lary.27209.

Wallace DV, Dykewicz MS, Bernstein DI, Blessing-Moore J, Cox L, Khan DA, Lang DM, Nicklas RA, Oppenheimer J, Portnoy JM, Randolph CC, Schuller D, Spector SL, Tilles SA. The diagnosis and management of rhinitis: an updated practice parameter. J Allergy Clin Immunol. 2008;122(2):S1–S84. https://doi.org/10.1016/j.jaci.2008.06.003.

Wang Y, Jin L, Liu SX, Fan K, Qin ML, Yu SQ. Role of nasal saline irrigation in the treatment of allergic rhinitis in children and adults: a systematic analysis. Allergol Immunopathol. 2020;48(4):360–7. https://doi.org/10.1016/j.aller.2020.01.002.

Welsh PW, Stricker WE, Chu CP, Naessens JM, Reese ME, Reed CE, Marcoux JP. Efficacy of beclomethasone nasal solution, flunisolide, and cromolyn in relieving symptoms of ragweed allergy. Mayo Clin Proc. 1987;62(2):125–34. https://doi.org/10.1016/s0025-6196(12)61882-5.

Yáñez A, Rodrigo GJ. Intranasal corticosteroids versus topical H1 receptor antagonists for the treatment of allergic rhinitis: a systematic review with meta-analysis. Ann Allergy Asthma Immunol. 2002;89(5):479–84. https://doi.org/10.1016/S1081-1206(10)62085-6.

Chapter 7
Subcutaneous and Sublingual Immunotherapy

Timothy Kaddis, Jonathan Jalali, Karishma Raju, Vivian Wang, and Joseph Yusin

Historical Perspective of Allergen Immunotherapy

Allergen immunotherapy, commonly known as allergy shots, is an effective treatment option for those who have been diagnosed with allergic rhinitis, asthma or atopic dermatitis. The idea of receiving injections that consist of allergen extracts made from environmental pollen originated from the pollen theory, introduced in the late 1800s and perfected by William Dunbar (Noon 1960).

Charles Blackley, a doctor who lived in Manchester, England, played a major role in developing and proving this theory. Dr. Blackley thought grass and other environmental pollens were the main culprit in triggering symptoms of allergic rhinitis. He placed pollen extract on a special skin test device that then was applied to a patient's skin, causing a pruritic, swollen red bump in patients with allergic rhinitis. His studies solidified the true cause of allergic rhinitis (Blackley 2021).

In the early 1900s, Dr. William Dunbar expanded on the pollen theory and offered a treatment option. He referred to pollen as "toxins." He produced an "antitoxin" by injecting the toxin into an animal. The animal's blood/serum was then extracted and prepared as a powder, ointment or fluid. He discovered that topical application of the antitoxin powder or ointment into nasal passages or subcutaneous injections of the antitoxin fluid into human subjects who suffered from allergic

T. Kaddis (✉) · J. Jalali · K. Raju · V. Wang · J. Yusin
Department of Medicine, David Geffen School of Medicine at UCLA, Los Angeles, CA, USA

VA Greater Los Angeles Health Care System, Los Angeles, CA, USA
e-mail: tkaddis@mednet.ucla.edu; JJalali@mednet.ucla.edu; KRaju@mednet.ucla.edu; Vivian.Wang@va.gov; Joseph.Yusin2@va.gov

M. Mahmoudi (ed.), *Treatment and Management of Allergic Rhinitis*,
https://doi.org/10.1007/978-3-031-88107-7_7

rhinitis prevented symptoms when exposed to environmental pollens. Dr. Dunbar manufactured this antitoxin and named it "Pollantin" (Bailey 1903).

During this time, Sir Almroth Wright, who originally developed a vaccine against typhoid fever founded the Saint Mary's Laboratory and Research Institute. There Dr. Leonard Noon was recruited to study the treatment of hay fever. He was the first to show repeated injections of grass pollen in patients with hay fever led to a decrease in symptoms when exposed to pollen. He worked closely with Dr. John Freeman, who later took over after the passing of Noon from tuberculosis, carrying out further studies showing the benefit of subcutaneous immunotherapy, similar to allergen immunotherapy given now (Cohen and Dworetzky 2002).

Over time, the idea of a toxin producing an antitoxin that was able to decrease hay fever symptoms was overrun by the idea of sensitization. Pioneered by such investigators as Dr. Karl Koessler, who hypothesized that instead of toxins, there were specific sensitizers within grass that caused the symptoms, and that repeated allergen injections would produce an antibody that could prevent the these pollen protein sensitizers from interacting with cells, leading to tolerance (Cooke 1915). This theory was later proven by Dr. Robert Cooke, one of the founders of the Allergy Immunology field, who concluded that with gradual introduction of allergen, an inhibiting substance, possibly an antibody, prevents the sensitized antibody from interacting with a cell that would lead to an allergic response (Cooke et al. 1935).

Despite being accepted and utilized for years, the first double-blind placebo-controlled study on allergen immunotherapy was not published until 1954 by Frankland, which confirmed the benefit of such therapy over placebo (Durham and Shamji 2023).

Mechanisms of Allergen Immunotherapy

Though the clinical practice of allergen immunotherapy (AIT) far predates the discovery of its mechanistic basis, several mechanisms have now been elucidated by which it induces immunologic tolerance to antigens, thereby improving symptoms of allergic rhinitis. Natural allergen exposure causes symptoms by inducing a pro-inflammatory response via Th2 cytokine signaling, resulting in IgE-mediated mast cell activation and eosinophil migration to tissues. On the contrary, AIT opposes these effects by activating pro-regulatory pathways.

Important pro-regulatory pathways underlying the efficacy of immunotherapy include activation of tolerogenic dendritic cells as well as peripheral regulatory T cells (Treg) which express IL-10, transforming growth factor-B (TGF-B), and IL-35 (Gueguen et al. 2016; Zimmer et al. 2012; Akdis et al. 1998; Francis et al. 2008; Bohle et al. 2007; O'Hehir et al. 2009; Shamji et al. 2019a). Central FOXP3+ Treg cells are induced as well. These T regulatory cells act via cytokine signaling and direct cell-cell interaction to, among other effects, induce B cell isotype class switching to IgG, IgA, which compete with IgE for allergen binding. This directly inhibits the formation of allergen-IgE complexes, reducing the IgE-mediated presentation of allergen to B cells and dendritic cells, as well as downstream activation of mast cells and basophils (Ling et al. 2004; Pilette et al. 1950; Shamji et al. 2019b). The relative importance of each of these mechanisms, as well discovery of novel aspects of regulatory mechanisms involved in AIT, remains an active area of research.

Subcutaneous Immunotherapy: Patient Selection, Preparation, and Administration

Patient Selection

In the United States, subcutaneous immunotherapy (SCIT) remains the most common form of inhalant allergen immunotherapy, owing to its well-established efficacy and safety. Nevertheless, risk benefit determination should be individualized for each patient based on the considerations below prior to initiation of an AIT regimen.

Age

SCIT has been long been safely administered to both adults and children. Though there is no absolute lower limit on age for this treatment, children under the age of 5 are uncommonly started on immunotherapy due to intolerance of repeated injections and inability to report reaction symptoms. Likewise, there is no consensus upper age limit for immunotherapy, as patient comorbidities are a more effective indicator of risks (Cox et al. 2011).

Comorbidities

The most significant comorbid medical conditions to consider in assessing patient risk are those which have the potential to adversely affect treatment of anaphylaxis with epinephrine. These include, but are not limited to, arrhythmias, coronary artery disease, hypertension, and cerebrovascular disease. Furthermore, concurrent use of β-blocker medications can inhibit response to epinephrine during anaphylaxis, and every effort should be made to consider alternatives to these medications in patients undergoing immunotherapy, if available. Though there has traditionally been concern regarding immunotherapy in patients with autoimmunity or immunodeficiency, increased risk in these patients has not been well established (Cox et al. 2011).

Pregnancy

Several studies of immunotherapy in pregnant women have not shown increased incidence of abortion, prematurity, congenital malformations, or other adverse outcomes. Therefore, patients undergoing immunotherapy who become pregnant during the maintenance phase of treatment are commonly continued at their current dose. However, due to concerns about the risk that severe adverse reactions may pose to a pregnant woman, fetus, or both, immunotherapy is not usually initiated or built-up during pregnancy. If a patient becomes pregnant during the buildup phase of immunotherapy, the decision of whether to discontinue treatment or continue at the last tolerated dose for the duration of pregnancy should be individualized and take into consideration the likelihood that the last tolerated dose is sufficient to be therapeutic (Metzger et al. 1978; Shaikh 1993).

Preparation and Administration of Subcutaneous Immunotherapy

Preparing SCIT Serum

Once a patient's sensitization profile has been established via skin prick or serum IgE testing, the prescribing allergist selects clinically significant allergens for which the patient will undergo immunotherapy. Effective maintenance doses are selected, which are unique to each allergen and usually range from 5 to 20 μg. Maintenance doses have been standardized for many major inhalant allergens, and suggested doses are available for most which have not been standardized to date. Maintenance doses of each allergen are then combined to form the maintenance concentrate that will be used to treat the patient. The maintenance concentrate is then diluted so that a careful titration or build-up process can be initiated, often starting at one thousandth or one ten thousandth of the maintenance concentration and increasing periodically until the full concentration is achieved (Cox et al. 2011).

Administering SCIT

Standard build-up schedules most commonly involve single weekly injections, after which a maintenance dose is achieved within 6–8 months. Maintenance injections are then given on a monthly basis. Accelerating this build-up process is often desirable for faster symptom relief and optimized patient convenience. Accelerated schedules range in duration from 1 to 3 days, referred to as "rush immunotherapy," to 4–8 weeks, referred to as "cluster immunotherapy." However, rush and cluster immunotherapy schedules have been associated with higher risk of systemic reactions, a risk which should be discussed with patients who desire accelerated build-up.

Efficacy and Duration of Subcutaneous Immunotherapy (SCIT)

Subcutaneous immunotherapy (SCIT) is a cornerstone treatment for allergic rhinitis, offering relief that goes beyond symptom management by addressing the underlying immune response. Unlike medications, which provide temporary relief and require consistent use, SCIT involves a series of injections that progressively desensitize the immune system to create lasting change. Over time, patients experience significant reductions in nasal congestion, sneezing, and other allergy symptoms, even during peak allergen exposure. This therapy has consistently demonstrated its ability to improve the quality of life for individuals whose allergies are resistant to conventional treatments.

SCIT has demonstrated consistent efficacy in numerous clinical trials, including significantly reduced symptom scores compared to placebo. Patients typically experience a 30–40% reduction in symptom severity and medication usage during treatment. Patients undergoing SCIT often report a reduced need for antihistamines, nasal sprays, and other medications, which not only simplifies their daily routines but also minimizes the side effects associated with long-term medication use. Additionally, SCIT has been shown to improve overall respiratory health, particularly in individuals with severe or poorly controlled allergic rhinitis, enabling them to enjoy outdoor activities and other environments that were previously intolerable.

One of the most remarkable aspects of SCIT is its potential for long-term effectiveness. After completing a typical treatment course of 3–5 years, many patients continue to experience relief from symptoms for years without additional therapy. This sustained benefit is attributed to the immune system's adaptation during the treatment period, which fosters a lasting state of tolerance to the allergens. In addition, early intervention, particularly in children, may further enhance these benefits by targeting immune development during a critical period. For some, the improvements are so significant that their allergic symptoms become minimal or even negligible in daily life.

The duration of SCIT therapy is a critical factor in achieving these lasting benefits. Research indicates that a minimum of 3 years is necessary to establish durable immune changes and ensure persistent symptom relief. This extended treatment period allows the immune system to undergo gradual and comprehensive reprogramming, transforming the body's response to allergens from overreactive to tolerant. Patients who complete the full course of therapy often find the investment in time well worth the substantial and enduring improvements in their allergic symptoms.

In conclusion, SCIT stands out as an effective and transformative therapy for allergic rhinitis. Its ability to provide significant, long-lasting relief and reduce reliance on medications makes it an invaluable option for individuals struggling with the burdens of refractory disease. By committing to the full duration of therapy, patients can achieve reduced symptom burden, medication use, and even remission of disease (Calderon et al. 2007; Durham et al. 1999; Penagos and Durham 2022).

Development of Sublingual Immunotherapy (SLIT)

Sublingual therapy is an excellent alternative for patients who are sensitized to ragweed, specific northern pasture grasses like Timothy grass, and dust mites. Importantly, it offers the convenience of being able to self-administer aeroallergen immunotherapy at home. The first randomized control trial involving sublingual immunotherapy dates back to 1986. Sublingual immunotherapy was first developed during this time as an alternative to subcutaneous immunotherapy with hopes that there would be less adverse effects, particularly less prevalence of anaphylaxis, with this modality (Aboshady and Elghanam 2014). Oral mucosa was a tactical target in pursuits of finding an alternative to subcutaneous immunotherapy. Oral mucosa is the center of frequent allergen exposure yet is not often a site of acute inflammation and allergic reaction, which suggest some degree of local immune tolerance. Oral mucosal tolerance involves the deletion or the functional inactivation of T cells by means of apoptosis or active inhibition by co-inhibitory receptors. It also involves the development of antigen-specific T cells that selectively suppress immune system activation by specific antigens (Min et al. 2023). Interestingly, only a few studies regarding the effect of sublingual immunotherapy on the T cell response exist, and they suggest that sublingual immunotherapy may work my modulating the TH2—biased allergic immune response (Brimnes et al. 2007).

Allergen immunotherapy, regardless of modality, yields increased production of T regulatory cells and inhibitory cytokines like interleukin-10. Additionally, there are decreases in allergen-specific immunoglobulin E. In patients receiving subcutaneous immunotherapy, the IgE-inhibitory activity is predominantly mediated by allergen-specific IgG-4, but for patients receiving sublingual immunotherapy this inhibition is primarily mediated by IgA1 or IgA2 (Durham and Shamji 2023). Because of this, within weeks of starting allergen immunotherapy, the production of many different specialized cell types including T cells, dendritic cells, eosinophils, mast cells and basophils is inhibited.

In a study by Brimnes et al. in which mice were sensitized by intraperitoneal injections of alum-adsorbed phleum pratense extract and then subsequently treated with SLIT, it was demonstrated that SLIT treatment can reduce allergic symptoms in a time- and dose-dependent manner. Eosinophilia and IgE levels in the nasopharyngeal lavage were reduced by more than 50% in the sensitized mice treated with SLIT (Brimnes et al. 2007).

Administration of Sublingual Immunotherapy (SLIT)

Sublingual immunotherapy can be administered in two different forms. The allergen extract can be prepared in a tablet or a drop formulation. The patient is instructed to keep the tablet or drop under the tongue for 1–3 min prior to swallowing. This allows for the antigen to be absorbed through the sublingual mucosa. The myeloid and Langerhans dendritic cells then detect the allergen and reduce the Th1 and Th2 immune responses through the secretion of different interleukins such as IL-10, IL-12, IL-27 and transforming growth factor-beta. Since the sublingual immunotherapy is not systemically administered, the allergen is less likely to be absorbed in the blood which subsequently results in decreased prevalence of systemic adverse effects such as anaphylaxis (Min et al. 2023).

Subcutaneous Immunotherapy (SCIT) Versus Sublingual Immunotherapy (SLIT) : A Comparison

In indirect meta-analysis comparing the efficacy of SLIT versus standard pharmacotherapy with intranasal corticosteroids and oral antihistamines, it was shown that SLIT revealed efficacy greater than oral antihistamines and comparable with intranasal corticosteroids (Durham and Shamji 2023). When specifically comparing the efficacy of SLIT versus SCIT, it has been indicated in previous randomized control trials that 3 years of consistent therapy with either sublingual or subcutaneous immunotherapy results in decreased seasonal rhinitis symptoms and decreased reliance on antiallergic medications that endured for at least 2 years after discontinuation. However, in a randomized clinical trial performed by Scadding et al. comparing the effects of treatment with grass pollen subcutaneous immunotherapy with grass pollen tablet sublingual immunotherapy, it was demonstrated that at year 1 subcutaneous immunotherapy was more effective than sublingual immunotherapy in reducing total nasal symptom scores after challenge. The study also demonstrated that, in contrast to 3 years of either treatment, 2 years of treatment was insufficient to maintain tolerance 1 year after stopping therapy (Scadding et al. 2017).

Moreover, it is important to keep in mind that currently the only forms of SLIT approved by the Food and Drug Administration are for dust mites, ragweed, and northern pasture grasses like Timothy grass. Additionally, the prevalence of systemic adverse reactions is lower with SLIT compared to SCIT. Therefore, assessing which modality of treatment is more appropriate for the patient should depend on the results of the patient's allergy testing, response to standard pharmacotherapy (i.e. oral antihistamines, nasal sprays), schedule flexibility and atopic comorbidities (Table 7.1).

Table 7.1 Comparison of subcutaneous and sublingual immunotherapy

Route	Subcutaneous immunotherapy (SCIT)	Sublingual immunotherapy (SLIT)
Allergen extract availability	Most major allergens	FDA approved tablets for: House dust mite Ragweed Northern pasture grasses
Efficacy	Well-established in placebo-controlled clinical trials for most major allergens	SLIT tablet products (listed above) well established in placebo-controlled clinical trials
Adverse reactions	Local reactions: Injection site swelling, erythema, irritation Systemic reactions: Urticaria Exacerbation of rhinitis or asthma symptoms Anaphylaxis	Local reactions: Oral pruritus Localized angioedema Systemic reactions: Eosinophilic esophagitis Anaphylaxis
Frequency	Build-up phase: Weekly Maintenance phase: Monthly Accelerated build-up protocols available	Daily
Duration	3–5 years	3–5 years
Setting of administration	All injections administered in clinic	Initial dose administered in clinic, self-administration at home thereafter

Ensuring the Safety of Administering Subcutaneous and Sublingual Immunotherapy

Subcutaneous Immunotherapy (SCIT)

Administration and Monitoring for Reactions

SCIT is recommended to be administered under medical supervision for all doses. It is standard practice to monitor patients for at least 30 min following each injection to observe for potential adverse reactions (Cox et al. 2011). The primary goal of SCIT is to safely complete the buildup phase and achieve the maintenance dose. However, during dose adjustments and even during the maintenance phase, patients may experience both local and systemic reactions.

Local reactions occur at the injection site and typically include redness, itching, and swelling. These symptoms can usually be managed with supportive care, such as topical corticosteroids, cool compresses, or oral antihistamines (Cox et al. 2011). Local reactions can also be minimized by pre-medicating with an oral antihistamine. If a patient experiences frequent large local reactions, the dose may be repeated or reduced during the buildup or maintenance phases. Although this adjustment does not guarantee the prevention of future local or systemic reactions, it is considered standard practice to improve patient tolerance and minimize discomfort.

The most serious systemic reactions usually occur within 30 min of the injection, which is why it is standard practice to observe patients during this time. Symptoms of systemic reactions can involve multiple organ systems and range in severity, from mild rhinitis or hives to life-threatening anaphylaxis. Staff must be trained to recognize these symptoms so patients can be treated immediately with epinephrine and other measures (Cox et al. 2011).

Delayed systemic reactions can also occur, however they are less common. These typically present 30 min or more after the injection and are usually less severe than immediate reactions. Biphasic systemic reactions can occur in rare cases, with a second phase of symptoms arising 2–24 after the initial reaction. The second phase is generally less severe but still requires monitoring and appropriate management (Cox et al. 2011; Confino-Cohen and Goldberg 2010).

It is recommended that all patients bring their epinephrine autoinjector to their immunotherapy appointments and keep it with them afterwards. This precaution ensures they are prepared to treat a delayed systemic reaction immediately, should one occur. Additionally, patients should be educated about the signs and symptoms of systemic reactions and how to self-administer epinephrine in an emergency.

SCIT Risk Management and Patient Considerations

To minimize the risk of severe reactions, staff responsible for administering immunotherapy should be trained in safety protocols. One common cause of systemic reactions is the administration of immunotherapy to the wrong patient. It is essential to verify the correct patient and the correct vial(s) before each injection. This verification process should include confirming two patient identifiers, such as name and date of birth. Additionally, at each visit, patients should be questioned about any reactions they may have experienced after their last injection to ensure any necessary adjustments are made.

Patients with stable asthma and a forced expiratory volume in 1 s (FEV1) of 70% or more are generally eligible for SCIT, provided there are no other significant comorbidities (Cox et al. 2011; Zuberbier et al. 2010). However, if a patient is experiencing an asthma exacerbation, immunotherapy should be deferred, and the exacerbation should be appropriately managed before resuming treatment. Special consideration should also be given to patients who are pregnant or taking beta-blockers, as these conditions may increase the risk of systemic reactions or complicate their management (Cox et al. 2011). In such cases, the risks and benefits of continuing immunotherapy should be evaluated, and dose adjustments may be necessary. Additionally, any new medical conditions or changes in the patient's health should prompt a reevaluation of their immunotherapy plan.

Sublingual Immunotherapy

Initial Dose Supervision and Home Administration
It is recommended that the first dose of sublingual immunotherapy (SLIT) be administered in the clinic under medical supervision, with the patient observed for 30 min afterward. This precaution ensures that any symptoms suggestive of an allergic reaction can be promptly addressed. If the patient tolerates the initial dose without issues, subsequent doses can be safely administered at home.

Studies have shown that SLIT is commonly associated with local symptoms, such as oral pruritus, while serious systemic side effects are rare (Burks 2020; Rodríguez-Pérez et al. 2008). Most patients tolerate the first dose well under medical supervision and can proceed with home administration. Local reactions, although often more intense at the start of therapy, tend to improve over time with continued treatment. However, some patients may experience significant local itching making them uncomfortable taking it at home without supervision. In these situations, SLIT may be a less suitable option for them, and switching to subcutaneous immunotherapy (SCIT) may be more appropriate.

Patient Education and Missed Dose Management for SLIT
All patients should be educated about systemic symptoms and prescribed an epinephrine autoinjector for home use in case of anaphylaxis. When taking SLIT tablets, patients should ensure their hands are clean and dry before touching the tablet. The tablet should be placed sublingually for at least 1 min or until fully dissolved. Patients should avoid eating or drinking for five minutes following administration.

If a patient misses a single dose, they can resume therapy without adjusting the dose. However, if they miss more than seven consecutive days, they should contact their allergist for guidance on restarting therapy. Premedication with antihistamines is not required prior to taking SLIT tablets. However, if antihistamines are part of the patient's existing allergic rhinitis or rhinoconjunctivitis regimen, they should continue their usual treatment.

Summary and Conclusion
Allergen immunotherapy (AIT) provides relief for patients suffering from allergic rhinitis by inducing several pro-regulatory pathways of the immune system and dampening the Th2 response to allergens. Both subcutaneous and sublingual forms of AIT have proven highly efficacious for allergic rhinitis and are safe options in appropriately selected patients.

References

Aboshady OA, Elghanam KM. Sublingual immunotherapy in allergic rhinitis: efficacy, safety, adherence and guidelines. Clin Exp Otorhinolaryngol. 2014;7(4):241–9.

Akdis CA, Blesken T, Akdis M, Wüthrich B, Blaser K. Role of interleukin 10 in specific immunotherapy. J Clin Invest. 1998;102(1):98–106.

Bailey FW. The present status of the Dunbar hay fever therapy. Laryngoscope. 1903;13(12):917–20.
Blackley CH. Experimental researches on the causes and nature of Catarrhus Æstivus. Legare Street Press; 2021. p. 238.
Bohle B, Kinaciyan T, Gerstmayr M, Radakovics A, Jahn-Schmid B, Ebner C. Sublingual immunotherapy induces IL-10-producing T regulatory cells, allergen-specific T-cell tolerance, and immune deviation. J Allergy Clin Immunol. 2007;120(3):707–13.
Brimnes J, Kildsgaard J, Jacobi H, Lund K. Sublingual immunotherapy reduces allergic symptoms in a mouse model of rhinitis. Clin Exp Allergy. 2007;37(4):488–97.
Burks AW, editor. Middleton's allergy: principles and practice. 9th ed. Edinburgh: Elsevier; 2020. p. 2.
Calderon MA, Alves B, Jacobson M, Hurwitz B, Sheikh A, Durham S. Allergen injection immunotherapy for seasonal allergic rhinitis. Cochrane Database Syst Rev. 2007;2007(1):CD001936.
Cohen S, Dworetzky M. The allergy archives: pioneers and milestones. J Allergy Clin Immunol. 2002;109(1):179–84.
Confino-Cohen R, Goldberg A. Allergen immunotherapy-induced biphasic systemic reactions: incidence, characteristics, and outcome: a prospective study. Ann Allergy Asthma Immunol. 2010;104(1):73–8.
Cooke RA. The treatment of hay fever by active immunization. Laryngoscope. 1915;25(2):108–12.
Cooke RA, Barnard JH, Hebald S, Stull A. Serological evidence of immunity with coexisting sensitization in a type of human allergy (hay fever). J Exp Med. 1935;62(6):733–50.
Cox L, Nelson H, Lockey R, Calabria C, Chacko T, Finegold I, et al. Allergen immunotherapy: a practice parameter third update. J Allergy Clin Immunol. 2011;127(1 Suppl):S1–55.
Durham SR, Shamji MH. Allergen immunotherapy: past, present and future. Nat Rev Immunol. 2023;23(5):317–28.
Durham SR, Walker SM, Varga EM, Jacobson MR, O'Brien F, Noble W, et al. Long-term clinical efficacy of grass-pollen immunotherapy. N Engl J Med. 1999;341(7):468–75.
Francis JN, James LK, Paraskevopoulos G, Wong C, Calderon MA, Durham SR, et al. Grass pollen immunotherapy: IL-10 induction and suppression of late responses precedes IgG4 inhibitory antibody activity. J Allergy Clin Immunol. 2008;121(5):1120–5.
Gueguen C, Bouley J, Moussu H, Luce S, Duchateau M, Chamot-Rooke J, et al. Changes in markers associated with dendritic cells driving the differentiation of either TH2 cells or regulatory T cells correlate with clinical benefit during allergen immunotherapy. J Allergy Clin Immunol. 2016;137(2):545–58.
Ling EM, Smith T, Nguyen XD, Pridgeon C, Dallman M, Arbery J, et al. Relation of CD4+CD25+ regulatory T-cell suppression of allergen-driven T-cell activation to atopic status and expression of allergic disease. Lancet Lond Engl. 2004;363(9409):608–15.
Metzger WJ, Turner E, Patterson R. The safety of immunotherapy during pregnancy. J Allergy Clin Immunol. 1978;61(4):268–72.
Min JY, Jee HM, Lee HY, Kang SY, Kim K, Kim JH, et al. The KAAACI guidelines for sublingual immunotherapy. Allergy Asthma Immunol Res. 2023;16(1):9–21.
Noon L. Prophylactic inoculation against hay fever. Historical document. Ann Allergy. 1960;18:287–91.
O'Hehir RE, Gardner LM, de Leon MP, Hales BJ, Biondo M, Douglass JA, et al. House dust mite sublingual immunotherapy: the role for transforming growth factor-beta and functional regulatory T cells. Am J Respir Crit Care Med. 2009;180(10):936–47.
Penagos M, Durham SR. Allergen immunotherapy for long-term tolerance and prevention. J Allergy Clin Immunol. 2022;149(3):802–11.
Pilette C, Nouri-Aria KT, Jacobson MR, Wilcock LK, Detry B, Walker SM, et al. Grass pollen immunotherapy induces an allergen-specific IgA2 antibody response associated with mucosal TGF-beta expression. J Immunol Baltim Md. 1950;178(7):4658–66.
Rodríguez-Pérez N, et al. Frequency of acute systemic reactions in patients with allergic rhinitis and asthma treated with sublingual immunotherapy. Ann Allergy Asthma Immunol. 2008;101(3):304–10.

Scadding GW, Calderon MA, Shamji MH, Eifan AO, Penagos M, Dumitru F, et al. Effect of 2 years of treatment with sublingual grass pollen immunotherapy on nasal response to allergen challenge at 3 years among patients with moderate to severe seasonal allergic rhinitis: the GRASS randomized clinical trial. JAMA. 2017;317(6):615–25.

Shaikh WA. A retrospective study on the safety of immunotherapy in pregnancy. Clin Exp Allergy J Br Soc Allergy. 1993;23(10):857–60.

Shamji MH, Layhadi JA, Achkova D, Kouser L, Perera-Webb A, Couto-Francisco NC, et al. Role of IL-35 in sublingual allergen immunotherapy. J Allergy Clin Immunol. 2019a;143(3):1131–42.

Shamji MH, Kappen J, Abubakar-Waziri H, Zhang J, Steveling E, Watchman S, et al. Nasal allergen-neutralizing IgG4 antibodies block IgE-mediated responses: novel biomarker of subcutaneous grass pollen immunotherapy. J Allergy Clin Immunol. 2019b;143(3):1067–76.

Zimmer A, Bouley J, Le Mignon M, Pliquet E, Horiot S, Turfkruyer M, et al. A regulatory dendritic cell signature correlates with the clinical efficacy of allergen-specific sublingual immunotherapy. J Allergy Clin Immunol. 2012;129(4):1020–30.

Zuberbier T, Bachert C, Bousquet PJ, Passalacqua G, Walter Canonica G, Merk H, et al. GA^2 LEN/EAACI pocket guide for allergen-specific immunotherapy for allergic rhinitis and asthma. Allergy. 2010;65(12):1525–30.

Chapter 8
Osteopathic Philosophy Applied to Rhinitis

Meghan Callahan, Remie Saab, Eshika Kohli, and Robert W. Hostoffer

Abbreviations

OMM	Osteopathic manipulative medicine
DO	Doctor of Osteopathic Medicine
MD	Medical Degree
A.T.	Andrew Taylor
GERD	GastroEsophageal Reflux Disease

Introduction

Osteopathic manipulative medicine (OMM) has become an increasingly common practice in modern medicine, and in many ways, it is what separates a Doctor of Osteopathic Medicine (DO) from their allopathic counterparts (MD). OMM is more than just a physical practice, but also a philosophy behind the way DO physicians

The authors Meghan Callahan, Remie Saab, Eshika Kohli, and Robert Hostoffer have been equally contributed to the research, development, and writing of this chapter.

M. Callahan (✉)
Lake Erie College of Osteopathic Medicine, Elmira, NY, USA
e-mail: mcallahan68657@med.lecom.edu

R. Saab · R. W. Hostoffer
Cleveland Medical Center, University Hospitals, Cleveland, OH, USA

E. Kohli
Lake Erie College of Osteopathic Medicine at Seton Hill, Greensburgv, PA, USA

M. Mahmoudi (ed.), *Treatment and Management of Allergic Rhinitis*,
https://doi.org/10.1007/978-3-031-88107-7_8

study and engage in medicine. The philosophy of Osteopathic Medicine is complex and virtuous.

Andrew Taylor (A.T.) Still, MD, DO, was a prominent physician in the midwestern United States during the nineteenth century. He found that medicine at this time did not address the entire scope of disease holistically. The focus of medicine at the time was not on using the body's natural processes to remedy itself. His initial philosophy was focusing on the interconnections of an individual's body, mind, and spirit. During his lifetime, his writings never included any description of manual medicine, but a description of his philosophy of medicine. His initial pronouncement of a physician treatment using the body, mind, and spirit, was later distilled into four tenets, and eventually, further delineated into osteopathic models (A.T. Still Biography n.d.; Still AT 1892) (Tables 8.1, 8.2, and 8.3).

Rhinitis is a clinical diagnosis that involves the presence of nasal symptoms such as sneezing, rhinorrhea, nasal congestion or itchiness, and cough. There are a wide range of etiologies behind this clinical picture, but most commonly patients suffer from allergic rhinitis. Allergic rhinitis falls into the range of disease processes known as atopy; a commonly allergic process mediated by IgE inflammation (Hruby and Hoffman 2007; Hughes and Nibbs 2018). The treatment of rhinitis—whether it be allergic or not—has not changed considerably as of recent years. The standard of treatment includes avoidance of triggers (commonly allergens) and intranasal corticosteroids and antihistamines (Dykewicz et al. 2020; Hannoodee and Nasuruddin 2024). As effective as these are, they do not rid patients of the entire disease and have significant side effects. Osteopathic philosophy will contribute to the overall resolution of rhinitis symptomology when coupled with the other treatment modalities.

The history of philosophy traces the development of human thought from ancient civilizations, modern times, exploring fundamental questions about existence, knowledge, values, reason, and the nature of reality. Beginning in the ancient world, with the pre-Socratic thinkers of Greece that progressed through the works of Socrates, Plato, and Aristotle, relayed the groundwork for Western philosophy. Today, philosophy continues to evolve integrating interdisciplinary approaches and addressing contemporary issues. Philosophers are individuals who ask questions about present mindsets or therapies (Patel et al. 2022). The philosopher constantly looks for improvement of their existence and others through questions. A.T. Still,

Table 8.1 The application of body, mind, and spirit to rhinitis

Body, mind, and spirit	Relation to rhinitis
Body	Physical touch with patients is an important aspect in a physical examination and serves as a touchstone communication.
Mind	Eye contact is essential in connecting with a patient during examination to ensure that the patient feels heard and understood.
Spirit	Patient trust is a core component of good health care. Utilizing the mind and body in coherence with spirit enables a healthcare provider to develop optimal patient trust.

From: Seffinger (2018)

Table 8.2 The application of the four osteopathic tenets to rhinitis

Osteopathic tenets	Relation to rhinitis
The body is a unit; the person is a unit of body, mind, and spirit.	The nasal passages that involve the pathology of rhinitis need to be thought of with respect to the remainder of the body attached. Systemic afflictions, as well as afflictions of other organs, may be a contributing cause to rhinitis and must be taken into consideration.
The body is capable of self-regulation, self-healing, and health maintenance.	When looking at rhinitis, thebody's ability to create immunoglobulins, cytokines, and chemokinesaid in thebody's healing capacity to fight the inflammatory effects involved in rhinitis.
Structure and function are reciprocally interrelated.	When evaluating for rhinitis, the bony structure of the nasal passages may obstruct the passageways and obstruct function. This can also be looked at from an immunological standpoint referring to immunoglobulins, cytokines, chemokines, structure, and reciprocal function.
Rational treatment is based upon an understanding of the basic principles of body unity, self-regulation, and the interrelationship of structure and function.	In this aspect, rhinitis forms a structural, immunological, and holistic approach which serves to resolve and/or diminish the inflammatory effects found in rhinitis.

From: Seffinger (2018)

Table 8.3 The application of the five osteopathic models to rhinitis

Osteopathic models	Relation to rhinitis
Biomechanical	This model merges the mechanical aspect of nasal passages with the biologic component of fighting pathogen in the scenario of rhinitis.
Respiratory-Circulatory	This model describes how obstructive processes of the nares can impact circulation and the venous and arterial flow through the nasal passages.
Neurological	This model emphasizes the role of different types of sensation (such as itch, pain, etc.) with rhinitis.
Metabolic-Energy	This model applies the role of soluble blood factors to rhinitis.
Behavioral	This model describes the way that the patient approaches and understands rhinitis, whether that is by frustration, anxiety, or pain.

From: Seffinger (2018), Giusti (2017)

MD, DO, was the one who questioned the modalities of medicine at the time and searched for new ways to find health. In this very way, he and his students may be considered physician philosophers (A.T. Still Biography n.d.).

A.T. Still, MD, DO, was born in Lee County, Virginia and he developed the philosophy of osteopathic medicine when he identified a lack of medical care for patients. In 1864, three of Still's children died from spinal meningitis. A.T. Still utilized this detrimental event in his life to further fuel his passion to pursue a new method to practice medicine (Still AT 1908). From 1853 to 1879, Still practiced orthodox medicine; however, after several years, Still began to use manipulative treatment in place of traditional medicine to treat various diseases. He realized that patients treated with manipulative medicine without the use of drugs would have the same or better outcomes than those treated with drugs. It is important to remember that most of the drugs that were available at that time are today considered as poisons such as arsenic, mercury, and procedures that are now archaic such as leeches and bleeding (Justiz Vaillant et al. 2024). Still had an interest in anatomy and utilized the musculoskeletal system as the center of his treatment methods. His motives included manipulation, but also philosophy that was mentioned in four of the books he wrote: *Autobiography of Andrew T. Still with a History of the Discovery and Development of the Science of Osteopathy*, *Philosophy of Osteopathy*, *The Philosophy and Mechanical Principles of Osteopathy*, and *Osteopathy Research and Practice.* His type of medicine was soon used by many of the students and development of a school of osteopathic medicine in Kirksville, Missouri (Brmi n.d.; Seffinger 2018). His choice of naming this new type of medicine as osteopathic (i.e. Doctor of Osteopathy) was used to differentiate it from the standard medical degree (MD), so that his medicine would not be usurped as did occur with homeopathy. In the following pages, we aim to further explore his philosophy in respect to rhinitis (Slocum 2010; Still AT 1910).

A.T. Still was one of the first to propose an approach that a physician should holistically be looking at the body, mind, and spirit (Table 8.1). In relation to the first component, the body, A.T. Still said,

> Osteopathy is based on the perfection of Nature's work. When all parts of the human body are in line, we have health. When they are not, the effect is disease. When the parts are readjusted, disease gives place to health. The work of the osteopath is to adjust the body from the abnormal to the normal, then the abnormal conditions give place to the normal and health is the result of the normal condition.

From our understanding, A.T. Still wanted to explain the importance of manipulating the body to guide its healing. When the body is not in line, there is no health. The purpose of a physical examination ofa patient is to understand why the patient may lack health. This is done using mechanisms such as touch and palpation to understand the patient and the problems they may be facing (Bordoni 2020; Giusti 2017).

The second component of Still's philosophy focuses on the mind. A.T. Still stated that, "Osteopathy… is the law of mind, matter, and motion." We believe that A.T. Still wanted to add an emphasis on engaging the mind when looking at the patient in his holistic approach. When the patient's mind is engaged, it can be observed through their body language, as seen through eye contact. Eye contact remains an important aspect of patient care as it ensures the patient feels understood, and can help elicit the patient's symptoms if it is used in a physical exam setting (Still AT 1908).

The third and final aspect to A.T. Still's philosophy focuses on the spirit.

A.T. Still added that,

> It is a scientific knowledge of anatomy and physiology in the hands of a person of intelligence and skill, who can apply that knowledge to the use of man when sick or wounded by strains, shocks, falls, or mechanical derailment or injury of any kind to the body.

This provides an explanation of the importance of applying the knowledge gathered by physicians. Although A.T. Still does not directly talk about spirit in this statement, his readings suggest that spirit is directly involved in the application of patient care to gain trust. Physicians must gain trust to ensure that the patient will comply with appropriate medication use and treatment for their own betterment (Tuscano et al. 2024).

The body, mind, and spirit come together cohesively to be applied to rhinitis. A.T. Still notes that, "All diseases are mere effects, the cause being a partial or complete failure of the nerves to properly conduct the fluids of life." Still's philosophy can be applied to rhinitis. In reference to rhinitis, the physical examination of the body's structure can be observed through the airflow through the nasal passages. In treating patients with rhinitis, the mind plays an important role in maintaining the patient's engagement through eye contact. Spirit can be observed by the trust that has developed between the physician and patient over time (Widdicombe 1997).

After Still's death, his philosophy gathered from his books was distilled into what is known today as the Tenets of Osteopathic Medicine. These are briefly described in Table 8.2. The first tenet states that the body is a unit that encompasses the body, mind, and spirit (Seffinger 2018). In the case of rhinitis, one cannot separate the structure of the nares from the rest of the body including blood flow and neurologic innervation. The systemic effects of disease in the body in a different anatomical location may impact the nasal passages. For example, when gastrointestinal reflux disease(GERD)is active, nasal congestion may be experienced, the nasal congestion will not be adequately treated using intranasal medications—but will only be resolved when the underlying cause, in this case GERD, is treated (Lin et al. 2015).

The second tenet claims that the body is capable of self-regulation, self-healing, and health maintenance. The body has a natural healing ability which includes the production of immunoglobulins, cytokines, and chemokines that work to fight pathogens and remodel, populate, or repopulate structures (Hannoodee and Nasuruddin 2024; Hughes and Nibbs 2018). These soluble blood factors can be used in either defensive or recuperative nature. Their secretion and transport require a liquid medium, like blood, and a highway, like arteries and veins, to distribute its protective and healing capabilities. The flow, in general, may be obstructed by musculoskeletal dysfunction preventing these capacities to be utilized. A.T. Still, MD, DO, realized that correcting the obstruction to flow may allow the body to heal itself via the rule of the artery. Although A.T. Still had no knowledge of these soluble factors, his observations suggested that something in the blood, when allowed to flow unobstructed, assisted in the healing of the patient.

The nasal passages are a very vascular structure. The protective and healing nature of the immune system often courses through these vascular structures. This flow allows for a balance of proper nasal function to ward off infection and/or heal the area from other insults.

The third tenet is that structure and function are reciprocally interrelated. The structure that Andrew Taylor Still, MD, DO, commonly referred to was the musculoskeletal system. At this time, he viewed the structure of the musculoskeletal system when appropriately aligned allowed for optimal and appropriate function of the body as a whole. More closely, this structure alignment allowed for blood flow and other soluble factors to protect and/or heal any compromised anatomic structure. On a cellular level, a disruption of a receptor structure on a cell surface will create a mismatch with its corresponding immunoglobulin, cytokine, or chemokine; this disruption will eventually cause a functional abnormality and immune response. This reality may also be realized intracellularly at a nuclear level (Hannoodee and Nasuruddin 2024; Hughes and Nibbs 2018). It is clear that an understanding of the previous three tenets, when used together, creates a framework for the understanding of pathology and to the subsequent search for health.

As a further distillation of his philosophy, a system of five models of Osteopathic care were developed (Table 8.3). In the first approach, the models described a biomechanical adjustment. This references the idea that the musculoskeletal system, when in dysfunction, may inhibit the motion of the soluble factors to destinations in the body that would require defense or repair (Paul et al. 2023; Remien et al. 2024). In the case of rhinitis, the evaluation of congestion and lymphatic flow or drainage patterns may demonstrate an obstruction that would limit resolution of nasal congestion, infection, or atopy.

The second model refers to the respiratory-circulatory process. This model addresses the fact that there are certain areas in the body that are referred to as diaphragms which may cause restriction to venous, arterial, and lymphatic flow when in dysfunction. These diaphragms of the upper respiratory tract are located at the thoracic inlet and thoracic outlet. In reference to rhinitis, these diaphragms will require evaluation, and when in dysfunction, to be relieved in order for appropriate drainage and/or passage of blood flow and lymphatic fluids to and from the upper respiratory tract.

The neurological model suggests that there must be an autonomic balance that will address neural reflex activity, remove facilitated segments, decrease afferent nerve signals, relieve pain. In reference to rhinitis, the evaluation for Chapman's reflexes in the upper respiratory areas may be resolved when in dysfunction and change the abnormal autonomic innervations. This change in sympathetic innervations will influence the mucus consistency, nasal congestion, and drainage routes of the nasal passages.

The metabolic model evaluates the self-regulatory and self-healing mechanisms to foster energy conservation by balancing the body's energy expenditure in exchange to enhance the immune system's function, endocrine function, and other organ function. In reference to rhinitis, the evaluation of musculoskeletal obstruction and correction will lead to improved immunological, endocrinological resources available for the improvement of the nasal environment.

The behavioral model aims to improve the biological, psychological, and social components of the health spectrum. In reference to rhinitis, the evaluation of the patient's emotional state, stressors in their lives, may have an influence on the type of systemic responses (immune, endocrine, and circulatory) required to keep a balance of health within the nasal passages.

Example Case

A 46-year-old male has had chronic rhinosinusitis over the last 5–6 years, which is coincided with obtaining a new pet, new apartment, job, and a move from a southern to a northern state. He complains of nasal congestion, sinus pressure, and post-nasal drainage. The symptoms are perennial, but clearly worse when he is laying flat. He also states that he is fatigued, and finds his sleep un-replenish able. To combat his fatigue, he has consumed several caffeinated beverages throughout the day. This has caused him some level of anxiety due to its effect on his work and free time.

His physical exam demonstrated fullness of his frontal and maxillary sinuses with application of pressure. His eyes demonstrated allergic shiners. His nasal passages were obstructed with very little space for airflow due to swollen nasalturbinates. The posterior pharyngeal wall showed marked cobblestoning. The remainder of his physical exam was unremarkable.

Rational

Body, Mind, and Spirit

During the physical exam, the physician makes contact by touch to the affected areas. In addition, the physician's conversation will delve into his personal life and habits while making eye contact throughout the exam. The patient-physician contact emphasizes a level of caring which produces a trust between the physician and patient.

Tenets

During the physical exam, the patient was examined with attention to the nasal passages, as not just a separate unit, but as a part of the whole body. This helped to define the patient's core problems, which was silent GERD, which produced both the nasal congestion and post-nasal drainage. By prompting a diet change, which eliminated caffeinated beverages, the patient was able to correct their nasal congestion and develop a better sleep pattern (Gardiner et al. 2023). This, over several weeks, resolved his fatigue, and subsequently, his anxiety. The structural abnormality of nasal congestion created a generalized dysfunction, but resolved when the structure was placed back into health.

Models

The biomechanical model is demonstrated by the production of gastric secretions producing the nasal congestion and post-nasal drainage. The nasal congestion found, due to the swollen turbinates, obstructed the function of the nasal passages, which would have resolved with attention to the other models and tenets. The neurological model can be noted from the sinus pressure, which was also resolved with the attention of the other models and tenets. The metabolic model can be observed from the inflammatory mediators that the gastric acid sensation produced in the nasal passages. The general observations of anxiety demonstrated the behavioral model within the patient's history, which was resolved with the appropriate dietary changes (Gelis et al. 2007; Hruby and Hoffman 2007).

Summary and Conclusion

Andrew Taylor Still, MD, DO's philosophy was one that suggested the evaluation of the entire body in attempt to find health. Further distillation of his philosophy into the tenets has aided the physicians to centralize the disturbance to health and models produced an outline of investigation. The utilization of this philosophy, the tenets, and the models helps the physician develop a more holistic approach to the disorder of rhinitis and the eventual development of a physician philosopher.

References

A.T. Still Biography. A.T. Still University. https://www.atsu.edu/museum-of-osteopathic-medicine/museum-at-still. n.d.; Accessed 11 June 2024.

Bordoni B. The five diaphragms in osteopathic manipulative medicine: myofascial relationships, part 1. Cureus. 2020;12(4):e7794. Published 2020 Apr 23. https://doi.org/10.7759/cureus.7794.

Brmi. History – Andrew Taylor still, MD, DO. Bioregulatory Medicine | BRMI Bioregulatory Medicine Institute. https://www.brmi.online/andrew-taylor-still. n.d.; Accessed 11 June 2024.

Dykewicz MS, Wallace DV, Amrol DJ, Baroody FM, Bernstein JA, Craig TJ, Dinakar C, Ellis AK, Finegold I, Golden DBK, Greenhawt MJ, Hagan JB, Horner CC, Khan DA, Lang DM, Larenas-Linnemann DES, Lieberman JA, Meltzer EO, Oppenheimer JJ, Rank MA, Shaker MS, Shaw JL, Steven GC, Stukus DR, Wang J, et al. A practice parameter update. J Allergy Clin Immunol. 2020;146(4):721–67. https://doi.org/10.1016/j.jaci.2020.07.007. Epub 2020 Jul 22

Gardiner C, Weakley J, Burke LM, et al. The effect of caffeine on subsequent sleep: a systematic review and meta-analysis. Sleep Med Rev. 2023;69:101764. https://doi.org/10.1016/j.smrv.2023.101764.

Gelis N, Prokopakis E, Helidonis E, Velegrakis G. Investigation of the relationship between allergic rhinitis and personality traits using semeiometry. Hippokratia. 2007;11(3):138–41.

Giusti R, editor. Glossary of osteopathic terminology. 3rd ed. Chevy Chase: American Association of Colleges of Osteopathic Medicine (AACOM); 2017.

Hannoodee S, Nasuruddin DN. Acute Inflammatory Response. In: StatPearls. StatPearls Publishing; 2024. http://www.ncbi.nlm.nih.gov/books/NBK556083/. Accessed 11 June 2024.

Hruby RJ, Hoffman KN. Avian influenza: an osteopathic component to treatment. Osteopath Med Prim Care. 2007;1:10. Published 2007 Jul 9. https://doi.org/10.1186/1750-4732-1-10.

Hughes CE, Nibbs RJB. A guide to chemokines and their receptors. FEBS J. 2018;285(16):2944–71. https://doi.org/10.1111/febs.14466.

Justiz Vaillant AA, Modi P, Jan A. Atopy. In: StatPearls [Internet]. Treasure Island (FL): StatPearls Publishing; 2024.

Lin YH, Chang TS, Yao YC, Li YC. Increased risk of chronic sinusitis in adults withgastroesophgeal reflux disease: a nationwide population-based cohort study. Medicine (Baltimore). 2015;94(39):e1642. https://doi.org/10.1097/MD.0000000000001642.

Patel SK, Srivastava S, Prajapati MKP. Greek Metaphysics and the Perspectives of Socrates, Plato and Aristotle in the Context of Physical Education. Integr J Res Arts Humanities. 2022;2(5):108–11. https://doi.org/10.55544/ijrah.2.5.17.

Paul NP, Galván AE, Yoshinaga-Sakurai K, Rosen BP, Yoshinaga M. Arsenic in medicine: past, present and future. Biometals. 2023;36(2):283–301. https://doi.org/10.1007/s10534-022-00371-y.

Remien K, Woo MJ, Vilella RC. Osteopathic manipulative treatment: lymphatic procedures. In: StatPearls. StatPearls Publishing; 2024. http://www.ncbi.nlm.nih.gov/books/NBK559051/. Accessed 11 June 2024.

Seffinger MA. Foundations of osteopathic medicine: philosophy, science, clinical applications, and research. Philadelphia: Wolters Kluwer; 2018.

Slocum PC. The Kirksville experience: where osteopathic medicine began. Mo Med. 2010;107(4):231–3.

Still AT. Autobiography of Andrew T. Still. Rev ed. Kirksville, MO: Published by the author, 1908. Distributed, Indianapolis: American Academy of Osteopathy.

Still AT. Osteopathy research and practice. Eastland Press; 1992. Originally published by the author; 1910.

Still AT. The philosophy and mechanical principles of osteopathy. Author, 1892. Then, Kansas City, MO: 1902. Reprinted, Kirksville, MO: Osteopathic Enterprises; 1986.

Tuscano SC, Haxton J, Ciardo A, Ciullo L, Zegarra-Parodi R. The revisions of the first autobiography of AT still, the founder of osteopathy, as a step towards integration in the american healthcare system: a comparative and historiographic review. Healthcare. 2024;12(2):130. https://doi.org/10.3390/healthcare12020130.

Widdicombe J. Microvascular anatomy of the nose. Allergy. 1997;52(40 Suppl):7–11. https://doi.org/10.1111/j.1398-9995.1997.tb04877.x.

Chapter 9
Osteopathic Drainage Techniques for Rhinitis

Olivia Humpel, Lauren Reinhold, Eshika Kohli, and Robert W. Hostoffer

Abbreviations

OMT	Osteopathic Manipulative Treatment
SPG	Sphenopalatine Ganglion

Introduction

Rhinitis is considered an inflammation of the nasal mucosa that can be allergic or no allergic in origin, characterized by symptoms such as rhinorrhea (infectious or non-infectious), post-nasal drainage, nasal congestion, sneezing, and pruritus (Wallace et al. 2008). Allergic rhinitis may show an engorgement of the nasal turbinates, which appear pale or violaceous. In contrast, viral rhinitis suggestserythematous turbinates. Simultaneous inflammation of the nasal cavity and sinus cavities lead to rhinosinusitis, which further involves mucosal erythema, discolored nasal and oro-pharyngeal secretions, and sinus tenderness on palpation (Seffinger 2018).

The authors Olivia Humpel, Lauren Reinhold, Eshika Kohli, and Robert Hostoffer have equally contributed to the research, development, and writing of this chapter.

O. Humpel (✉)
Lake Erie College of Osteopathic Medicine, Bradenton, FL, USA
e-mail: ohumpel29834@med.lecom.edu

L. Reinhold · R. W. Hostoffer
Cleveland Medical Center, University Hospitals, Cleveland, OH, USA

E. Kohli
Lake Erie College of Osteopathic Medicine at Seton Hill, Greensburg, PA, USA

M. Mahmoudi (ed.), *Treatment and Management of Allergic Rhinitis*,
https://doi.org/10.1007/978-3-031-88107-7_9

Parasympathetic over activity leads to increased nasal, lacrimal, and submandibular secretions. Cranial, cervical, and thoracic somatic dysfunctions may be evident, along with facial, glossopharyngeal, and vagus nerve dysfunction. The observation of somatovisceral reflexes suggests that somatic stimuli in these regions modulates visceral function and could impact sympathetic vasomotor tone (Seffinger 2018). Sympathetic preganglionic fibers arising from the upper thoracic and superior cervical ganglia innervate the sinuses. Structural defects or somatic dysfunction to the surrounding structures along this pathway may impact sympathetic tone and affect the health of the nasal mucosa via segmental facilitation (Nishida et al. 2015).

Somatic dysfunction of the upper ribs, upper thoracic spine, and clavicle may similarly impede lymphatic flow from the nose and sinuses. Lymphatic fluid from the head and neck enters central circulation near the subclavian and internal jugular veins (Seffinger 2018).

The earliest osteopathic technique for lymphatic drainage was the thoracic pump, developed by Dr. Earl Miller in 1920 (Chikly 2005). The thoracic pump technique was described as a direct method to relieve venous and lymphatic stasis and restoring circulation. Throughout the early twentieth century, lymphatic research was furthered by osteopaths Dr. Frederic Millard, Dr. William Galbreath, and Dr. Frank Chapman; the latter referred to the profound importance of the lymphatic aspects of disease of bony, muscular, or infectious origin (Chikly 2005).

Osteopathic approach to sinus and eustachian tube dysfunction incorporates lymphatic treatments, managing the most central or proximal obstruction first. Opening of the thoracic inlet, followed by doming of the diaphragm in cases of distal lymphatic congestion and respiratory abnormalities, are necessary for initial management. Facial effleurage, sphenopalatine ganglion (SPG) manipulation, ear tug, auricular drainage, mandibular drainage of Galbreath, cervical chain drainage, and suboccipital release may be implemented in a stepwise manner in both inpatient and outpatient clinical settings (Wu et al. 2020) (Table 9.1, Figs. 9.1, 9.2, 9.3, 9.4, 9.5, 9.6, 9.7, 9.8, and 9.9). This chapter provides an in-depth introduction into the osteopathic techniques for drainage, aiming to improve the symptoms of rhinitis.

Lymphatic treatment may be used in a rhinitis patient with signs of congestion. The focus of the treatment should be the most central obstruction. This includes an obstruction beginning in the head and neck or any thoracic or rib somatic dysfunctions. Treatment of the thoracic inlet is necessary prior to lymphatic techniques. Individuals with congestion distal to the diaphragm or with associated respiratory abnormalities also benefit from doming of the diaphragm. Lymphatic osteopathic manipulative treatment (OMT) may be performed in a stepwise manner: facial effleurage of the frontal and maxillary sinuses, SPG manipulation, ear tug, auricular drainage, mandibular drainage of Galbreath, cervical chain drainage, and suboccipital release (Wu et al. 2020) (Table 9.1, Figs. 9.1, 9.2, 9.3, 9.4, 9.5, 9.6, 9.7, 9.8, and 9.9).

Myofascial release of the thoracic inlet allows the physician to therapeutically assess the fascial continuum as the hand position contacts the bony anchors of the inlet (Table 9.1 and Fig. 9.1). The patient may be seated or supine, with the physician standing directly behind or seated at the head of the table, respectively. The physician's hands are placed atop the patient's shoulders, with thumbs pointing

Table 9.1 Treatment protocol for rhinitis patient

Figures	Lymphatic sequence	Treatment goal
1	Myofascial release of thoracic inlet	Enhance lymphatic drainage
2	Supine direct doming of diaphragm	Enhance mobility of diaphragm to improve lymphatic drainage
3	Frontal sinus effleurage	Improve mucociliary clearance and lymphatic drainage of head, ears, nose, and throat
4	Maxillary sinus effleurage	Improve mucociliary clearance and lymphatic drainage of head, ears, nose, and throat
5	Ear tug	Mobilize underlying fascia and temporal bone to open the eustachian tubes
6	Auricular drainage	Resolve fluid stasis of the middle ear and augment lymphatic drainage from the ear to the nose
7	Mandibular drainage (Galbreath)	Promote lymphatic drainage
8	Cervical chain drainage	Improve circulation in the ears, nose, and throat
9	Suboccipital release	Improve circulation and increase venous and lymphatic drainage to decrease edema
10	Sphenopalatine ganglion (figure not shown)	Enhance stabilization of the air ducts and decrease nasal obstruction

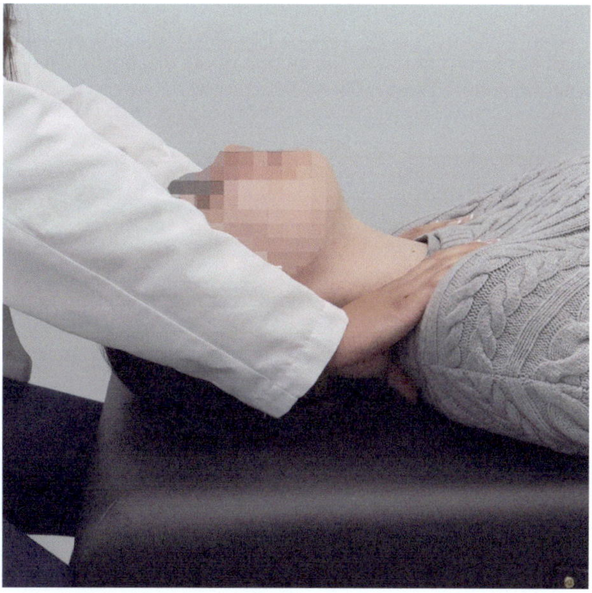

Fig. 9.1 Myofascial release of thoracic inlet. In this image, the patient is supine with the physician seated at the head of the table. The physician's hands are placed atop the patient's shoulders, with thumbs posteriorly towards the spinous processes of C7 and T1. The third and fourth fingers contact the first and second ribs anteriorly, superior to the clavicle. In this position, fascial motion patterns are assessed

posteriorly towards the spinous processes of C7 and T1. The third and fourth fingers contact the first and second ribs anteriorly, superior to the clavicle. In this position, the physician's hands relax and the palms rest on the patient's shoulders. Fascial motion patterns are assessed simultaneously in both hands. The physician must

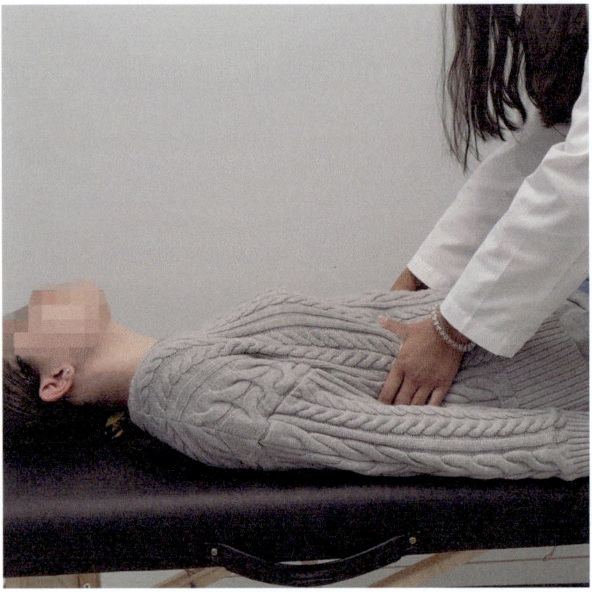

Fig. 9.2 Supine direct doming of diaphragm. The patient lies supine with knees bent. The physician places both hands on the anterolateral aspect of the inferior border of the ribs, with thumbs medial to the costal margins and directed to the xiphoid process. The patient is instructed to perform one full respiratory cycle. Upon exhalation, the physician's thumbs press posteriorly and slightly superior to follow the motion of the diaphragm. During inhalation, the physician resists anterior motion. These motions are repeated for several respiratory cycles

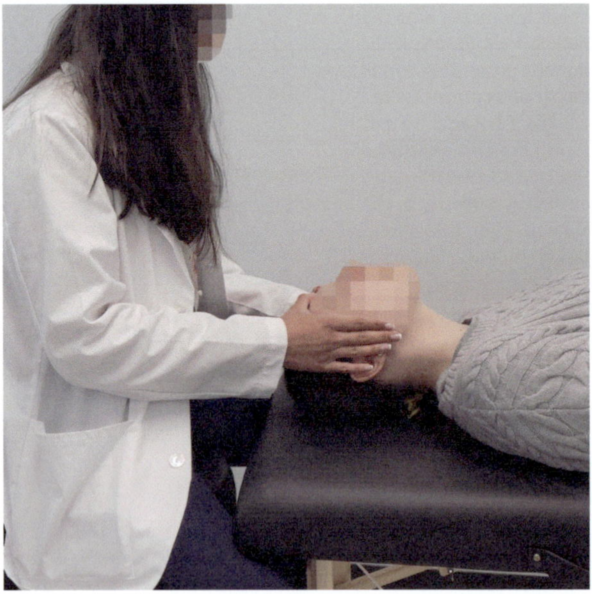

Fig. 9.3 Frontal sinus effleurage. The patient should be supine with the physician seated at the head of the table. To treat the frontal sinuses, the physician's thumbs are placed side by side at the center of the forehead and direct pressure is applied laterally towards the temples. At the lateral edge of the temporal fossa, the thumbs are directed inferiorly to the zygoma. This cycle is repeated six to eight times

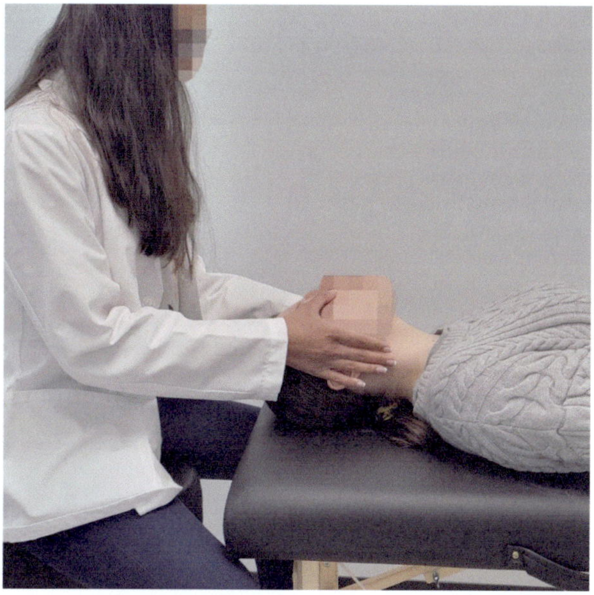

Fig. 9.4 Maxillary sinus effleurage. For the maxillary sinuses, the same technique as frontal sinus effleurage is used. The physician places their thumbs on either side of the nasal folds and used direct pressure along the maxilla

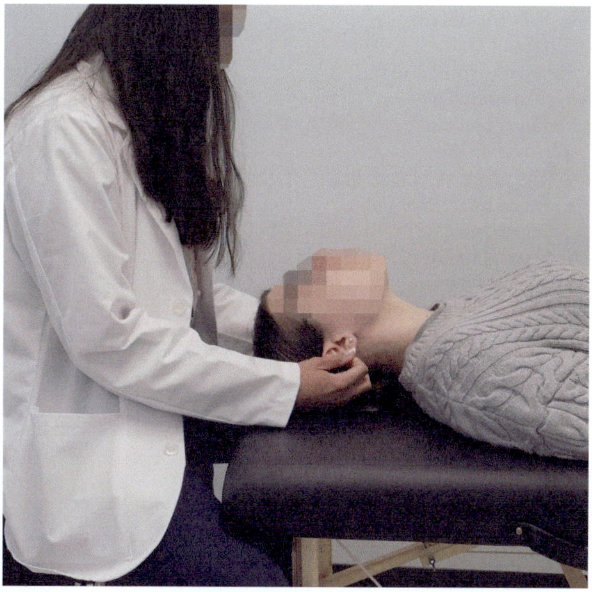

Fig. 9.5 Ear tug. The physician is seated behind the supine patient at head of the table. The physician gently grasps the pinnae bilaterally and applies equal posterolateral traction to open the eustachian tube

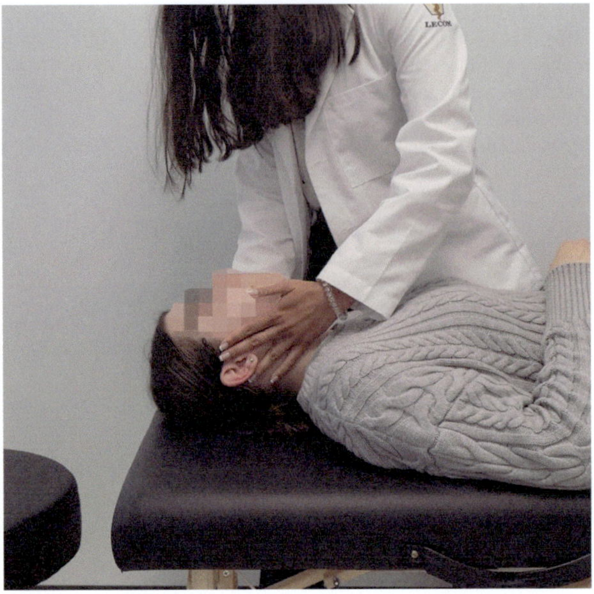

Fig. 9.6 Auricular drainage. The patient remains supine, and the physician uses their treatment hand to form a "V" with the third and fourth digits that is placed inferior to the external auditory canal. The opposite hand stabilizes the patient's head. The physician uses a firm, but gentle, pressure to perform small circular movements in a clockwise movement several times, followed by counterclockwise movements

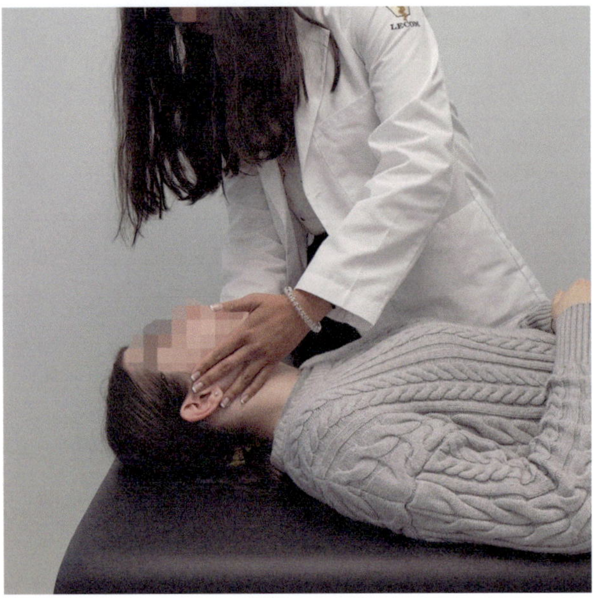

Fig. 9.7 Mandibular drainage of Galbreath. This technique is similar to the auricular drainage technique, but it is performed on the mandible. The technique is performed bilaterally on a supine patient. The physician places their contralateral thumb, index finger, and middle finger slightly above the upper jaw, while the physician's ipsilateral hand is used for stabilization. The patient is instructed to relax their jaw, and the physician applies gentle medial and caudad traction towards the opposite ear for 3–4 s before releasing

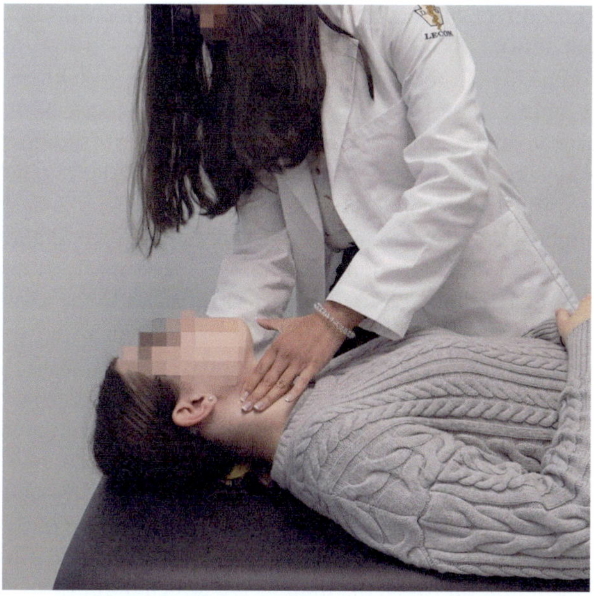

Fig. 9.8 Cervical chain drainage. The physician is seated at the head of a supine patient. The physician rotates the patient's head away from the side of treatment and the patient's head would be slightly flexed. The physician's thumb is placed on the anterior margin of the sternocleidomastoid in the inferior neck. The physician applies several slow, firm strokes along the inferior sternocleidomastoid, towards the clavicle. Further, the physician moves to the superior portion of the SCM at the top of the mastoid process (as pictured), and the stroking motion is repeated inferiorly for several cycles. Pressure to the carotid bodies should be avoided throughout the procedure

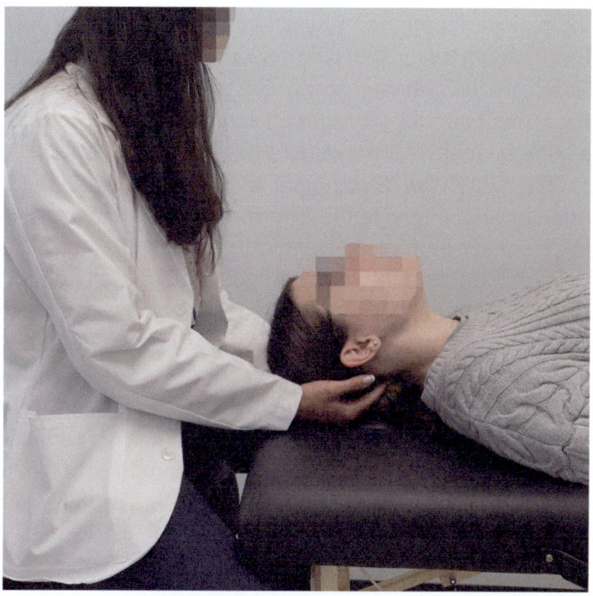

Fig. 9.9 Suboccipital release. With the patient supine, the physician places the finger pads of digits two through five in the patient's suboccipital sulcus bilaterally. The physician's elbows move medially with lateral traction placed on the suboccipital tissues. A gentle tractionis applied to the occiput until a release is felt

follow a direct or indirect approach with both hands for three subsequent respiratory cycles (Seffinger 2018).

To directly dome the diaphragm, the patient lies supine with knees bent to soften the abdomen (Table 9.1 and Fig. 9.2). The physician places both hands on the anterolateral aspect of the inferior border of the ribs, with thumbs medial to the costal margins and directed to the xiphoid process. The patient is instructed to perform one full respiratory cycle. Upon exhalation, the physician's thumbs press posteriorly and slightly superior to follow the motion of the diaphragm. During inhalation, the physician resists anterior motion. These motions are repeated for further exhalation and inhalation, and it is performed through several respiratory cycles. The physician may reassess for improvement by sensing decreased resistance under the thumbs in all phases of respiration (Seffinger 2018).

To facilitate drainage of the frontal and maxillary sinuses with effleurage, the patient should be supine with the physician seated at the head of the table (Table 9.1 and Figs. 9.3 and 9.4). The effleurage technique may be described as "milking", with direct pressure applied over the sinuses and gradually increased in a rhythmic motion. To treat the frontal sinuses, the physician's thumbs are placed side by side at the center of the forehead and are pulled laterally towards the temples. At the lateral edge of the temporal fossa, the thumbs are directed inferiorly to the zygoma. This cycle is repeated six to eight times. For the maxillary sinuses, the same technique is applied with the physician's thumbs beginning on either side of the nasal folds and sweeping laterally along the maxilla (DiGiovanna et al. 2020).

To perform the ear tug technique, the physician is seated behind the supine patient at head of the table, gently grasping the external ears bilaterally (Table 9.1 and Fig. 9.5). The physician applies equal posterolateral traction to open the eustachian tube.

Auricular drainage may be performed bilaterally (Table 9.1 and Fig. 9.6). With the patient supine, the physician's treatment hand forms a "V" with the third and fourth digits that is placed inferior to the external auditory canal. The opposite hand stabilizes the patient's head. The physician uses a firm, but gentle pressure to perform small circular movements in a clockwise movement several times, followed by a counterclockwise movement (Seffinger 2018).

The Galbreath technique, or mandibular drainage, is similar to the auricular drainage technique, but it is performed on the mandible (Table 9.1 and Fig. 9.7). The technique is performed bilaterally on a supine patient. The physician places their contralateral thumb, index finger, and middle finger (to the side of treatment) slightly above upper jaw, while the physician's ipsilateral hand adds stabilization. The patient is instructed to relax their jaw, and the physician applies gentle medial traction towards the opposite ear for 3–4 s before releasing (Seffinger 2018).

Cervical chain drainage involves effleurage of the anterior and posterior cervical chains (Table 9.1 and Fig. 9.8). This technique requires the physician to be seated at the head of a supine patient. It is important to note that pressure to the carotid bodies should be avoided throughout the procedure. The physician rotates the patient's head away from the side of treatment, and the patient's head may be flexed manually, or a pillow may be used to help facilitate drainage. The physician's thumb is placed on the anterior margin of the sternocleidomastoid in the inferior neck. The physician applies several slow, firm strokes along the inferior sternocleidomastoid, towards the clavicle. Next, the physician moves to the superior portion of the SCM at the top of the mastoid process, and the stroking motion is repeated inferiorly for several cycles (Seffinger 2018). This technique may be repeated along the posterior margin of the SCM and can be performed bilaterally. The physician must be careful not to apply pressure to the carotid arteries.

Suboccipital decompression, or suboccipital release, attempts to balance the suboccipital and occipito-atlantal tissues as they relate to the superior cervical ganglion and vagus nerve (Table 9.1 and Fig. 9.9). With the patient supine, the physician places the finger pads of digits two through five in the patient's suboccipital sulcus bilaterally. The physician's elbows move medially with lateral traction placed on the suboccipital tissues. A gentle traction, matching the resistance of the tissues, is applied to the occiputuntil a release is felt (Seffinger 2018).

Another method of treatment for rhinitis includes using OMT of the SPG (Kalamir et al. 2013) (Table 9.1). To complete this technique, the patient is placed in a supine position and the physician is seated beside the patient, contralateral to the side being treated. The physician stabilizes the patient's head by placing the palm of their cephalad hand in contact with the patient's vertex. Following, the physician asks the patient to open their mouth and shift their mandible laterally toward the treatment side. Simultaneously, the physician uses their caudad hand to apply pressure to the SPG. The physician does this by gently ascending their fifth digit of their caudad hand along the alveolar process of the maxilla to reach the pterygoid process. Once the pterygoid process has been located, the physician moves their finger cephalad and medial towards the SPG. The physician remains in this position until they feel release of the external pterygoid muscle. Once the physician feels a release, the physician will continue to move medial and cephalad into the pterygopalatine fossa to reach the SPG. The physician applies light pressure to the SPG with the pads of their fifth finger until they note tissue release. OMT for the SPGcan be applied to both sides, so it will be repeated on the contralateral side.

Case 1: Allergic Rhinitis

A 25-year-old male, known to have seasonal rhinitis to tree, grass, and ragweed presents during regional season with rhinorrhea, nasal and ear pruritis, and watery eyes. He experiences his symptoms only outdoors. He has utilized multiple nasal and ocular topical medication along with oral antihistamines with minimal relief.

His physical examination demonstrated a watery clear nasal discharge without turbinate edema. His conjunctiva is injected with tearing. His ear canals were clear.

Osteopathic Manipulative Treatment

Myofascial release of thoracic inlet
Supine direct doming of diaphragm
Ear tug
Auricular drainage
Cervical chain drainage
Suboccipital release

Case 2: Non-allergic Sinus Congestion and Rhinitis

A 40-year-old-female has had perennial sinus pressure particularly during the change of seasons. The pressure and fullness are located above the frontal and maxillary areas. There has been some nasal congestion with mild postnasal drainage. There is no pruritus. She has utilized multiple nasal steroids and oral decongestants that supply minimal relief.

Her physical examination demonstrated open nasal passages without drainage. Her conjunctival areas are without injection.

Osteopathic Manipulative Treatment

Myofascial release of thoracic inlet
Supine direct doming of diaphragm
Cervical chain drainage
Sphenopalatine ganglion manipulation

Case 3: Eustachian Tube Dysfunction and Rhinitis

A 50-year-old-female has had decreased hearing. She senses a "garbage can over the head" effect with vocalization. She has pain that radiates from the ear lobes bilaterally down to the angle of the jaw. She has had this sensation for several months with an unknown onset.

Her physical examination demonstrated nasal congestion with pale atrophic turbinates. The ears show no disturbance to the tympanic membranes and the canals were without cerumen. She has tried multiple nasal steroids and antihistamines and oral decongestants without relief.

Osteopathic Manipulative Treatment

Myofascial release of thoracic inlet
Supine direct doming of diaphragm
Ear tug
Auricular drainage
Mandibular drainage (Galbreath)
Cervical chain drainage
Suboccipital release

Summary and Conclusions

Rhinitis is a nasal process in response to noxious stimuli. Symptoms may include rhinorrhea, nasal pruritis, nasal congestion, sinus pressure and postnasal drainage. Such symptoms maybe disabling when involving sleep or work. Although environmental controls may benefit the individual, such controls may not resolve the symptoms completely. Medications may provide relief, but side effects can appear such as sedation or nasal irritation.

Osteopathic methods can provide significant relief for rhinitis, particularly when other modalities fail. The addition of an osteopathic protocol for rhinitis can be added easily into clinical practice. Further research is required to understand varying methods of osteopathic treatment for other respiratory disorders.

Techniques

References

Chikly BJ. Manual techniques addressing the lymphatic system: origins and development. J Am Osteopath Assoc. 2005;105(10):457–64.

DiGiovanna EL, Phykitt DE, Ferris MT. Chapter 111: HEENT applications. In: An osteopathic approach to diagnosis and treatment. 4th ed. Lippincott,. Williams & Wilkins; 2020. p. 527–37.

Kalamir A, Graham PL, Vitiello AL, Bonello R, Pollard H. Intra-oral myofascial therapy versus education and self-care in the treatment of chronic, myogenous temporomandibular disorder: a randomised, clinical trial. Chiropr Man Therap. 2013;5(21):17. https://doi.org/10.1186/2045-709X-21-17.

Nishida Y, Sopchak MM, Jackson MR, et al. Effect of select osteopathic manipulative treatment techniques on patients with acute rhinosinusitis. Am Acad Osteopath J. 2015;25(3):12–30.

Seffinger MA. Foundations of osteopathic medicine: philosophy, science, clinical applications, and research. Philadelphia: Wolters Kluwer; 2018.

Wallace DV, Dykewicz MS, Bernstein DI, et al. The diagnosis and management of rhinitis: an updated practice parameter. J Allergy Clin Immunol. 2008;122(suppl 2):S1–S84. https://doi.org/10.1016/j.jaci.2008.06.003.

Wu SS, Graven K, Sergi M, Hostoffer R. Rhinitis: the osteopathic modular approach. J Osteopath Med. 2020;120(5):351–8. https://doi.org/10.7556/jaoa.2020.054.

Chapter 10
The Use of Chapman Reflexes in the Diagnosis and Treatment of Rhinitis

Marija J. Rowane, Jessica Wilson, Eshika Kohli, Kate McDonough, and Robert W. Hostoffer

Abbreviations

OMM	Osteopathic Manipulative Medicine
CRs	Chapman reflexes
OMT	Osteopathic Manipulative Treatment
HEENT	head, eyes, ears, nose, throat

Introduction

Osteopathic Manipulative Medicine (OMM) considers anatomy and pathophysiology in the application of non-invasive, manual therapy, to improve structure and function of biomechanical, lymphatic, and neuroendocrine mechanisms. (Kuchera & Kuchera 2012; Wu et al. 2018a; Wu et al. 2018b; Wu et al. 2020; DiGiovanna et al. 2020; Nelson & Allgeier 2015), The interrelationship of the lymphatic and nervous systems with somatic and physiologic processes was first proposed in early osteopathic practice (Capobianco 2020; Fossum et al. 2018). The founder of

M. J. Rowane (✉)
Oklahoma State University Medical Center, Tulsa, OK, USA
e-mail: mrowane@okstate.edu

J. Wilson
Case Western Reserve University/ University Hospitals Cleveland Medical Center, Cleveland, OH, USA

E. Kohli
Lake Erie College of Osteopathic Medicine at Seton Hill, Greensburg, PA, USA

K. McDonough · R. W. Hostoffer
Allergy/Immunology Associates, Inc., Mayfield Heights, OH, USA

M. Mahmoudi (ed.), *Treatment and Management of Allergic Rhinitis*,
https://doi.org/10.1007/978-3-031-88107-7_10

osteopathic medicine, Andrew Taylor Still, MD, DO, recognized that "all diseases are mere effects and the cause being a partial or complete failure of the nerve to properly conduct the fluids of life." Still attributed dysfunctional tissue cells to inadequate capillary, lymphatic, and intercellular fluid circulation and, therefore, applied this concept to facilitate lymphatic drainage in his techniques (Deason 1940).

Frank Chapman, DO re-addressed this early understanding of the lymphatic system in 1901, after noticing positive clinical outcomes from direct, gentle manipulation of indurated "groin glands" and associated glands of the medial thighs, in a patient with severe adenitis (Fossum et al. 2018). Maurice Pilgrim, MD's 1903 proposal that mechanical stimulation of reflex centers influences bodily fluids and lymphatic drainage, in *Mechanical Vibratory Stimulation: Its Theory and Application in the Treatment of Disease*, inspired Chapman to further investigate "gangliform contracted lymphoid tissue nodules." Chapman's 1929 text, entitled *Lymphatic reflexes: a specific method of osteopathic diagnosis and treatment*, mapped over 200 "neurolymphatic points" and associated these with visceral and neuroendocrine glands. Charles Owens, DO, Chapman's brother-in-law and colleague at the American School of Osteopathy, communicated the concept of Chapman reflexes (CRs) to the osteopathic community after Chapman's death (Capobianco 2020; Fossum et al. 2018). Owens' *Mechanical Manipulation and Reflexes in the Treatment of Disease* (1940) explained these viscerosomatic tissue reflexes as a correspondence between visceral dysfunction secondary to local lymphatic stasis and tissue texture changes at a body surface point.

The historical definition of CRs have since evolved to the most updated description: "a system of reflex points that present as predictable anterior and posterior fascial tissue texture abnormalities…assumed to be reflections of visceral dysfunction or pathology" (Giusti 2017). Approximately 50 anterior and posterior CRs are recognized today (Capobianco 2020), based on the 200 neurolymphatic reflexes Chapman mapped over a century ago, with the "neuro" reflexes mediated by the autonomic nervous system and "lymphatic" reflexes involving all vasculature and affected by the sympathetic nervous system (Fossum et al. 2018). Visceral inflammation, spasm, or distention leads to dysfunction or disease, manifested as a palpable somatic clue (Kuchera & Kuchera 2012; Capobianco 2020). Facilitated spinal cord segments, such as T1 through T4 of the head, eyes, ears, nose, and throat (HEENT) region, transmit this reflex, propagating sympathetic outflow as somatic and/or visceral efferent responses. These sympathetic efferent impulses that traverse the cervical sympathetic chain ganglion produce somatic dysfunction, which may be manifested as specific myofascial tender points, such as CRs (Kuchera & Kuchera 2012).

Pathophysiology

A comprehensive approach to patient care considers the relationship of anatomical structure and physiological function and the body's inherent healing capacity (Wu et al. 2018a; Rowane & Evans 2019). Lymphatic vasculature of the upper respiratory tract drains from the nose, sinuses, and pharynx to the submandibular and retropharyngeal nodes, through the deep cervical lymphatic vessels, and then returns to venous circulation (Nelson & Allgeier 2015), a system that is impaired in rhinitis and other upper respiratory tract conditions. Rhinitis is an inflammatory immunologic reaction of the nose and paranasal sinuses, instigated by infections (viral or bacterial), allergens (food or inhalants), or irritants (chemical or mechanical) (Wu et al. 2018a; Wu et al. 2020). Lymphocytes secrete cytokines in these inflammatory reactions, such as helper T-cell type 2 recruiting interleukin (IL) 4, IL-5, and IL-13 in allergic rhinitis versus interferon γ, IL-6, IL-8, monocyte chemoattractant protein 1, granulocyte-macrophage colony-stimulating factor, and IL-10 involved in viral rhinitis (Wu et al. 2020). Inflammation of the lymphatic system modulates T-cell lymphocyte populations and function, precipitating nasal mucosal edema, excess mucous production, and decreased ciliary motility that may pervade peripheral structures (Wu et al. 2018a; Wu et al. 2020). Congenital or acquired anatomical anomalies, such as nasal polys or septal deviation, augment nasal obstruction and poor airway clearance. The engorgement of nasal mucosa by venous and lymphatic congestion contributes to the symptomatology of rhinitis or other upper respiratory conditions. Symptoms include but are not limited to rhinorrhea, epistaxis, dyspnea, pain, and sinus pressure. Recurrent infections and structural changes, such as mucous membrane thickening and ciliary dysfunction, develop from chronic inflammation, preventing adequate airway clearance and mucosal function (Wu et al. 2018a).

Acute or chronic nasal passage inflammation alters sympathetic nerve discharge, precipitating cranial, cervical, and upper thoracic tissue texture changes (Wu et al. 2018a). Cervical soft tissue hypertonia and range of motion restrictions; localized points of tenderness and tissue texture changes corresponding to CRs; increased nasal, lacrimal, and submandibular gland sections from parasympathetic hyperactivity; and facial, glossopharyngeal, and vagus nerve dysfunction are among osteopathic physical examination findings relevant to rhinitis (Kuchera & Kuchera 2012; Nelson & Allgeier 2015; Kuchera 2012; Harakal 1981). The viscerosomatic reflex patterns precipitating tissue texture changes, range of motion restrictions, and tenderness offer a practical diagnostic tool, supporting the diagnosis of upper respiratory conditions. The intensity of these viscerosomatic reflex tissue texture changes reflect the severity of associated visceral dysfunctions, offering additional diagnostic information (Nelson & Allgeier 2015).

Modulation of these HEENT viscerosomatic reflexes have the potential to inhibit or augment lymphatic drainage and to alleviate clinical symptoms (Wu et al. 2020). CRs in the suboccipital, cervical spine, clavicular, and upper thoracic regions target HEENT viscerosomatic reflexes associated with rhinitis (Table 10.1, Fig. 10.1a, b). Osteopathic Manipulative Treatment (OMT) offers a complementary tool in the comprehensive management of patients with rhinitis and other upper respiratory conditions (Kuchera & Kuchera 2012; Wu et al. 2018a; Wu et al. 2018b; Wu et al. 2020; Kuchera 2012; Harakal 1981; Hoyt 1990; Pintal 1989; Schmidt 1982). Gentle hands-on manipulation targeting associated viscerosomatic reflexes, as employed with CRs for example, provides a safe, non-pharmacologic approach to alleviating symptoms of rhinitis and potentially augmented the efficacy of other therapies (Nelson & Allgeier 2015).

Table 10.1 Chapman reflex topographical locations and visceral relationships of the head, eyes, ears, nose, throat, and lungs

Viscera	Chapman reflex location: Anterior	Chapman reflex location: Posterior	Associated infection(s) or disease(s)
Eye	Lateral aspect of surgical humeral neck	Lateral subocciput, posterior to mastoid process	Autoimmune (e.g. Sjogren), infectious conjunctivitis, keratoconjunctivitis sicca, ulceration
Ear	Superior surface of proximal clavicle, at intersection with first rib	C1 TP	Mastoiditis, otitis media with effusion, otitis externa, vertigo, tinnitus
Nasal sinus	Inferior surface of proximal clavicle, at intersection with first rib	C1 inferior articular process (i.e. midway between SP and TP, at articulation between adjacent vertebral segments)	Allergic or non-allergic rhinitis, chronic rhinosinusitis with or without nasal polyposis, epistaxis
Other sinuses	Superior surface of proximal second rib	C2 inferior articular process	Frontal, ethmoid, sphenoid, and/or maxillary sinusitis
Pharnyx	Superior surface of first rib, at intersection with clavicle	C2 inferior articular process	Pharyngitis (e.g. Streptococcal, viral), retropharyngeal abscess
Tonsils	First ICS, at sternal border	C2 inferior articular process	Tonsillitis (infectious mononucleosis), obstructive sleep apnea, peritonsillar abscess
Larynx	Superior surface of second rib, proximal to sternum	C2 inferior articular process	Aphonia, laryngitis, laryngomalacia, laryngotracheobronchitis (croup)
Bronchus	Second ICS, proximal to sternum	T2 lamina (i.e. midway between SP and TP)	Bronchitis, tracheitis
Upper lung	Third ICS, proximal to sternum	T3 lamina	Aspiration, pneumonia, tuberculosis
Lower lung	Fourth ICS, proximal to sternum	T4 lamina	Asthma, pneumonia

Adapted from Capobianco (2020), Fossum et al. (2018), and Kuchera and Kuchera (2012)
Abbreviation: *TP* transverse process, *SP* spinous process, *ICS* intercostal space

Diagnosis

CRs may be applied as a diagnostic tool in patients with HEENT symptoms, to identify the focal point of viscerosomatic dysfunction, among previously identified CRs in the suboccipital, cervical spine, clavicular, and upper thoracic regions

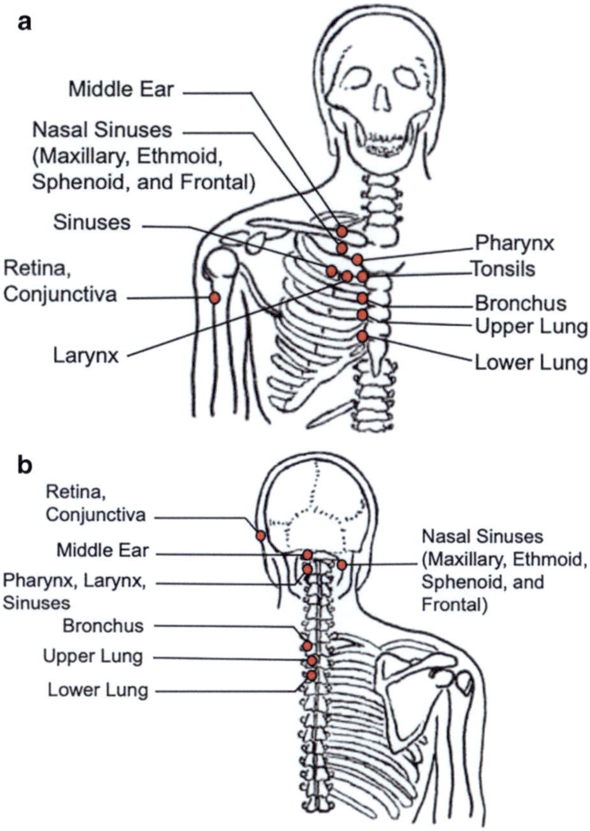

Fig. 10.1 (**a**) Anterior Chapman reflexes. (**b**) Posterior Chapman reflexes

(Table 10.1). CRs are palpable on physical exam as edematous, "shotty," or "fibro-spongy" tender tissue texture changes, often located in deep fascia or periosteum (Capobianco 2020; Fossum et al. 2018). Their variable dimensions range from the size of a pinhead to an almond, also comparable to a grain of rice, tapioca bead, or pea. Tenderness upon palpation ranges from slightly painful to nearly unbearable (Fossum et al. 2018). The intensity, or degree of tenderness on palpation, is reflective of the acuity of the involved viscera, such that a high pain level reported on palpation suggests an acute process, versus a diminished sense or lack of pain implies chronic, marked involvement. Chronic CRs are often "ropy" or "stringy" gangliform contractions, whereas acute CRs are typically found to be edematous and boggy (Capobianco 2020). History and other physical exam or structural findings guide the clinical significance of these CRs (Kuchera & Kuchera 2012).

The examiner directly contacts these sites with their index finger pad, while the patient is supine or seated, and elicits enough pressure to compress the skin to the periosteum of the rib, clavicle, or other bone surface (Kuchera & Kuchera 2012). Anterior CRs are traditionally identified first in diagnosis, given their more dispersed anatomical location and less tenderness on direct palpation, compared to their posterior CR counterparts. However, both anterior and posterior CRs must be present for a diagnosis (Table 10.1, Fig. 10.1a, b) (Capobianco 2020; Fossum et al. 2018). Anterior HEENT CRs are predominantly localized to the superior thoracic cage, supraclavicular or intercostal spaces (Table 10.1, Fig. 10.1a). Anterior CR identification is reinforced by diagnosis of associated posterior CRs (Fig. 10.1b). HEENT-associated posterior CRs are appreciated in the neck and upper cervical spine, primarily in the occipital and suboccipital regions (Table 10.1, Fig. 10.1b). Most posterior CRs along the cervical spine are localized midway between the spinous and transverse processes, on the lamina, as well as halfway the distance to the proximate inferior vertebrate, at the inferior articular process (Kuchera & Kuchera 2012).

CRs overlap with other systems of tissue texture abnormalities, such that topographical location comparative analyses of these points reported high correlation between acupuncture points and associated anterior (71%) and posterior (93%) CRs (Kuchera 2012). Other tissue texture abnormalities include myofascial trigger points, counterstrain tender points, fibromyalgia syndrome points as defined by the American College of Rheumatology, and acupuncture points. CRs are distinguished from their counterparts, as viscerosomatic tissue reflexes involving somatic dysfunction in the ganglion, paraspinal tissues, or cranial referral site of discrete viscera or glands. For example, Washington et al. identified a statistically significant relationship between pneumonia and associated CRs in hospitalized patients. A comprehensive diagnostic approach to CRs encourages differentiation from other somatic point systems, considering its discrete pathophysiology, associated signs and symptoms, and clinical implications (Fossum et al. 2018).

Treatment

CRs may be used selectively from a diagnostic perspective or considered for treatment. CRs are treated with direct rotatory stimulation for multiple seconds to minutes, 20–90 seconds on average, until the localized tissue texture tenderness and restriction or edema resolve (Fig. 10.2) (Kuchera & Kuchera 2012; Fossum et al. 2018). A gentle but firm rotatory movement is found to be most effective for the eye and ear, whereas a gentle rotatory movement is advised for the nasal, throat, and bronchial CRs (Fossum et al. 2018). Deep, firm rotary movement is suggested for the upper and lower lung. This specific rotatory stimulation may be applied to anterior and/or posterior CRs. Alternative OMT techniques, such as soft tissue, myofascial release, or balanced ligamentous tension, may be considered for application to regions involving CRs, as an alternative or additional step. After treatment of posterior CRs, anterior CRs are reassessed and, if tissue texture changes remain, gentle rotatory stimulation to the anterior CRs is applied (Kuchera & Kuchera 2012).

Application of OMT techniques to the HEENT region is contraindicated, when the patient presents with acute cranial nerve palsy, radiculopathy, diplopia, dysarthria, hypoxia, or ataxia, for example, that require immediate medical

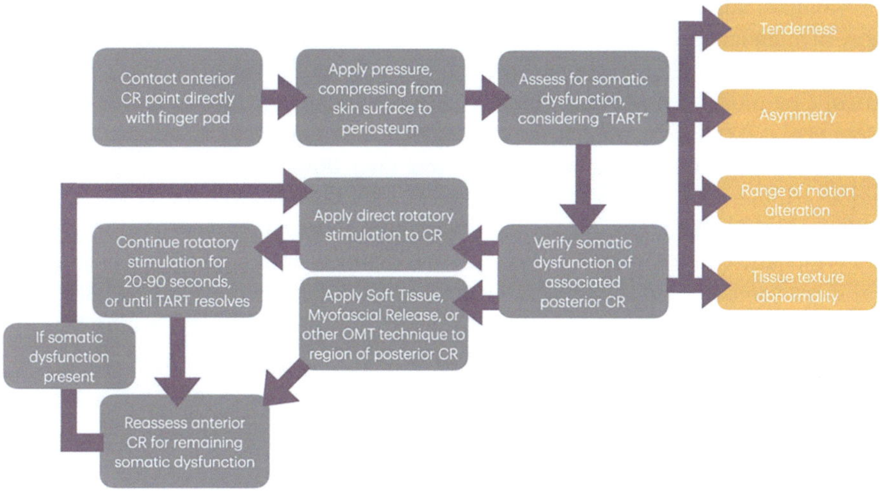

Fig. 10.2 Approach to CR diagnosis and treatment

intervention (Rowane & Evans 2019). History of a recent cerebrovascular accident or intracranial hemorrhage, severe rheumatoid arthritis, or intolerance with prior manual therapies should also be ruled-out, before OMT application (Kuchera & Kuchera 2012). Manipulation should be avoided at sites of active cutaneous infection, fracture, laceration, tumor, or pathologic bone disease (Rowane & Evans 2019).

Clinical Application

Limited studies investigated the clinical correlation of CRs. Washington et al. (2003) identified a statistically significant relationship between CRs and pneumonia in hospitalized patients. Few publications analyzed outcomes from OMT intervention limited to CRs. Lines et al. (1990) demonstrated significant improvement in forced vital capacity, from pre- to post-treatment, after application of CRs and soft tissue OMT techniques, in a cohort of 30 asymptomatic patients, including 5 patients with a history of asthma or bronchitis. Mannino (1978) reported decreased serum aldosterone levels for at least 36 hours after treated adrenal posterior CRs. A randomized control pilot trial, involving 25 females with polycystic ovary syndrome, found that 12 consecutive weeks of OMT intervention, including rib-raising and manipulation of CRs, improved post-exercise systolic blood pressure and heart rate recovery duration, as well as slightly lowered free testosterone levels (Davis et al. 2020). These studies are limited in sample size but demonstrated the efficacy of CRs in enhancing physiologic function (Washington et al. 2003; Lines et al. 1990; Mannino 1978; Davis et al. 2020).

Multiple animal models supported the proposed mechanism of CRs that application of manual techniques to stimulate fluid flow subsequently improved tissue repair processes and homeostasis. Intermittent pulsation pressure to the ventral thorax of a rat model demonstrated increased lymphatic uptake in peripheral tissues, in Dery et al. (2000). Dog models conducted by Knott et al. (2005) and Downey et al. (2008) demonstrated enhanced net thoracic duct flow from thoracic pump techniques. Hodge et al. (2007) measured significantly increased leukocyte counts from catheterized thoracic ducts in another dog model. These animal models modulated the lymphatics with direct manipulation and demonstrated subsequent physiological improvement (Dery et al. 2000; Knott et al. 2005; Downey et al. 2008; Hodge et al. 2007). The osteopathic literature necessitates more studies evaluating the clinical outcomes of OMT interventions, such as CRs (Wu et al. 2020).

Utilization in Rhinitis

A comprehensive approach to rhinitis management not only involves medical management, such as intranasal corticosteroids and antihistamines, oral antihistamines, and allergen-specific immunotherapy and biologics, and considers surgical management, if applicable, but also integrates patient education, environmental controls, and manual techniques, such as OMT.

Case Presentation

A 45-year-old female, with past medical history of allergic rhinitis, mild persistent asthma, and recent acute sinusitis, presented for an acute visit to the allergy/immunology clinic concerning persistent postnasal drip. The patient recently completed a 14-day course of doxycycline, with a prednisone taper, for acute sinusitis. Fever and yellow-green nasal discharge resolved within the first several days of antibiotics. Frontal, nasal, and maxillary sinus pressure, supra- and infra-ocular pressure, bilateral ear pressure, and postnasal drip improved since onset of illness. The patient was maximizing use of intranasal corticosteroid and antihistamine nasal sprays and sinus rinses. The review of systems was notable for mild bilateral ear pressure, nasal congestion and postnasal drip. The physical examination revealed mild bilateral tympanic membrane effusion without erythema and mild (1+) bilateral nasal turbinate edema. Osteopathic structural exam findings of somatic dysfunction included suboccipital muscle hypertonicity, cervicothoracic myofascial restriction, upper thoracic (T1–4) paraspinal hypertonicity, and a tender point at the inferior surface of the proximal clavicle, at its intersection with the first rib, consistent with

Table 10.2 Osteopathic Manipulative Treatment techniques to facilitate lymphatic drainage

Technique	Indications
Thoracic inlet release	Improve ROM of the first rib, cervicothoracic junction, and related fascia
Venous sinus drainage	Increase balance in dural membranes and CSF flow
Occipital-atlantal decompression	Increase OA ROM, reduce posterior headache, decreases nociceptive input from regional structures
Facial sinus pressure (effleurage Craniocervical)	Enhance fluid drainage of local head and/or neck structures
Galbreath Technique (mandibular drainage)	Drain the Eustachian Tube
Thoracic paraspinal inhibition	Improve ROM of the upper thoracics
Chapman's reflexes	Identify and treat viscerosomatic tender points, improving blood flow and enhancing medication distribution by decreasing sympathetic tone

an anterior CR. The corresponding posterior CR for the nasal sinus was identified at the C1 inferior articular process (i.e. midway between SP and TP, at the articulation between adjacent vertebral segments), as per Table 10.1 and Fig. 10.1a,b. Gentle application of circular pressure released these tender points, as per Fig. 10.2. The release of these points produced a positive clinical relief for the patient. Other OMT techniques, as demonstrated in Table 10.2, were applied with associated symptomatic benefit.

Summary and Conclusion

CRs are among multiple OMT techniques that offer a non-invasive, non-pharmacologic approach to optimizing rhinitis management (Kuchera & Kuchera 2012; Wu et al. 2018a; Wu et al. 2018b; Wu et al. 2020). These localized viscerosomatic tissue texture changes provide diagnostic information, suggesting the involved viscera, and serve as a simple target for direct manipulation (Capobianco 2020; Fossum et al. 2018). Many animal models and clinical studies suggest the influence of manipulation on immune pathophysiology, lymphatic circulation, and the autonomic nervous system (Washington et al. 2003; Lines et al. 1990; Mannino 1978; Davis et al. 2020; Dery et al. 2000; Knott et al. 2005; Downey et al. 2008; Hodge et al. 2007). More studies are indicated to specifically investigate CRs' mechanism of action and clinical significance. CRs of HEENT region may serve as diagnostic and therapeutic tools to complement or enhance standard medical management of rhinitis and associated conditions.

References

Capobianco JD. Chapter 22: Chapman's reflex points. In: DiGiovanni EL, Amen CJ, Burns DK, editors. An osteopathic approach to diagnosis and treatment. 4th ed. Lippincott: Williams & Wilkins; 2020. p. 94–102.

Chapman F. Lymphatic reflexes: a specific method of osteopathic diagnosis and treatment. Frank Chapman; 1929.

Davis SE, Hendryx J, Menezes C, et al. Weekly osteopathic manipulative treatment to improve measures of sympathetic tone in women with polycystic ovary syndrome: a randomized, controlled pilot study. J Am Osteopath Assoc. 2020;120(5):310–21. https://doi.org/10.7556/jaoa.2020.051.

Deason WJ. Body fluids – the original osteopathic concept: the influences behind Dr. Still's theories as revealed in his writings and interviews. Osteopath Prof Part I. 1940;7(7):9–11, 43–46; Osteopath Prof Part II. 1940;7(8):20–23, 43–45.

Dery MA, Yonuschot G, Winterson BJ. The effects of manually applied intermittent pulsation pressure to rat ventral thorax on lymph transport. Lymphology. 2000;33(2):58–61.

DiGiovanna EL, Phykitt DE, Ferris MT. Chapter 111: HEENT applications. In: DiGiovanni EL, Amen CJ, Burns DK, editors. An osteopathic approach to diagnosis and treatment. 4th ed. Lippincott: Williams & Wilkins; 2020. p. 527–37.

Downey HF, Durgam P, Williams AG Jr, et al. Lymph flow in the thoracic duct of conscious dogs during lymphatic pump treatment, exercise, and expansion of extracellular fluid volume. Lymphat Res Biol. 2008;6(1):3–13.

Fossum C, Kuchera ML, Devine WH, Wilson KL. 40E: a modern approach to chapman reflex points. In: Seffinger MA, et al., editors. Foundations of osteopathic medicine: philosophy, science, clinical applications, and research. 4th ed. Wolters Kluwer; 2018. p. 966–80.

Giusti R, editor. Glossary of osteopathic terminology. educational council on osteopathic principles. Chevy Chase: American Association of Colleges of Osteopathic Medicine; 2017.

Harakal JH. Manipulative treatment for acute upper-respiratory diseases. Ost Ann. 1981;9(7):30–37.

Hodge LM, King HH, Williams AG Jr, et al. Abdominal lymphatic pump treatment increases leukocyte count and flux in thoracic duct lymph. Lymphat Res Biol. 2007;5(2):127–33.

Hoyt WH III. Current concepts in management of sinus disease. J Am Osteopath Assoc. 1990;90(10):913–919.

Knott EM, Tune JD, Stoll ST, et al. Increased lymphatic flow in the thoracic duct during manipulative intervention. J Am Osteopath Assoc. 2005;105(10):447–56.

Kuchera ML. Counterstrain: Differential Diagnosis of Myofascial Points. In: Myers HL, ed. Clinical Application of Counterstrain, Compendium Edition. Osteopathic Press; 2012:20–28.

Kuchera ML, Kuchera WA. Osteopathic considerations in HEENT disorders. Greyden Press; 2012.

Lines DH, McMilan AJ, Spehr GJ. Effects of soft tissue technique and Chapman's neurolymphatic reflex stimulation on respiratory function. J Aust Chiropr Assoc. 1990;20(1):17–22.

Mannino JR. The application of neurological reflexes to the treatment of hypertension. J Am Osteopath Assoc. 1978;79:225–31.

Nelson KE, Allgeier J. Chapter 24: the patient with an upper respiratory infection. In: Nelson KE, Glonek T, editors. Somatic dysfunction in osteopathic family medicine. 2nd ed. Wolters Kluwer Heath/American College of Osteopathic Family Physicians; 2015.

Owens C. Mechanical manipulation and reflexes in the treatment of disease. Charles Owen; 1940.

Pilgrim MF. Mechanical vibratory stimulation. Lawrence Press; 1903.

Pintal WJ, Kurtz ME. An integrated osteopathic treatment approach in acute otitis media. J Am Osteopath Assoc. 1989;89(9):1139–1141.

Rowane MP and Evans P. Basic Musculoskeletal Manipulation Skills: The 15-Minute Office Encounter. 2nd ed. American Academy of Osteopathy; 2019.

Schmidt IC. Osteopathic manipulative therapy as a primary factor in the management of upper, middle, and pararespiratory infections. J Am Osteopath Assoc. 1982;81(6):382–388.

Washington K, Mosiello R, Venditto M, et al. Presence of Chapman reflex points in hospitalized patients with pneumonia. J Am Osteopath Assoc. 2003;103:479–83.

Wu SS, Hostoffer RW, Gibbons K, Shaw HH, Shaw MB. 48A(1): osteopathic considerations in patients with head, eyes, ears, nose, and throat disorders. In: Seffinger MA, et al., editors. Foundations of osteopathic medicine: philosophy, science, clinical applications, and research. 4th ed. Wolters Kluwer; 2018a. p. 1386–404.

Wu SS, Hostoffer RW, Gibbons K, Shaw HH, Shaw MB. 48A(2): rhinosinusitis. In: Seffinger MA, et al., editors. Foundations of osteopathic medicine: philosophy, science, clinical applications, and research. 4th ed. Wolters Kluwer; 2018b. p. 1404–11.

Wu SS, Graven K, Sergi M, Hostoffer R. Rhinitis: the osteopathic modular approach. J Am Osteopath Assoc. 2020;120(5):351–8. https://doi.org/10.7556/jaoa.2020.054.

Index

M. Mahmoudi (ed.), *Treatment and Management of Allergic Rhinitis*,
https://doi.org/10.1007/978-3-031-88107-7